# EXECUTIVE SUMMARY

## BACKGROUND

Traumatic brain injury (TBI) is a common condition, especially among military members. Twelve to 23 percent of service members returning from Operations Enduring Freedom, Iraqi Freedom, and New Dawn (OEF/OIF/OND) experienced a TBI while deployed. Although various criteria are used to define TBI severity, the majority of documented TBI events among OEF/OIF/OND service members may be classified as mild in severity, or mTBI, according to the definition used by the Veterans Health Administration and Department of Defense (VA/DoD).

While some researchers suggest most individuals recover within three months of an mTBI, others estimate that 10 to 20 percent of individuals continue to experience post-concussive symptoms (e.g., headaches, dizziness, balance problems) beyond this time fame. This estimate may be higher among OEF/OIF service members given the frequency of multiple TBI events, concomitant mental health conditions such as depression and posttraumatic stress disorder (PTSD), and other factors unique to combat deployments. As such, deployment-related mTBI is a significant issue for the VA, as patients who report ongoing mTBI symptoms may require the attention from a range of health care professionals. This evidence synthesis review will be used by the VHA TBI Advisory Committee to develop strategies to identify those at-risk for long-term mTBI effects, inform clinical practice, determine resource allocation, and identify future research priorities.

The key questions were:

Key Question #1. For Veteran/military populations, what is the prevalence of health problems (such as pain, seizure disorders, headaches, migraines, and vertigo), cognitive deficits, functional limitations (such as employment status, changes in marital status/family dynamics), and mental health symptoms (such as PTSD and depression) that develop or persist following mTBI?

Key Question #2. What factors affect outcomes for Veteran/military patients with mTBI? Key Question 2A: For Veteran/military populations, are there pre-injury (premorbid) risk/protective factors (e.g., pre-injury mental health factors, genetic factors, or prior concussions) that affect outcomes for mTBI? Key Question 2B: For Veteran/military populations, are there post-injury risk/protective factors (e.g., PTSD) that affect outcomes for mTBI?

Key Question #3. What is the resource utilization over time for Veteran/military patients with mTBI?

## METHODS

We searched Medline, PsychINFO and Cochrane Register of Controlled Trials (OVID), from database inception to October 3, 2012. We adapted the search strategy developed by the World Health Organization (WHO) Collaborating Centre for Neurotrauma Prevention, Management and Rehabilitation Task Force for a recent systematic review of prognosis after mTBI, and we included terms to identify articles specific to Veterans and military personnel. We obtained additional articles from systematic reviews, reference lists of pertinent studies, reviews, editorials, and by consulting clinical and research experts in the area of mTBI.

We included studies reporting outcomes in Veterans or military personnel who had suffered an mTBI using a case definition consistent with definitions in the VA/DoD Clinical Practice Guideline for Management of Concussion/Mild Traumatic Brain Injury. Reviewers trained in the critical analysis of literature assessed the titles and abstracts for relevance, and retrieved full-text articles for further review. We compiled a narrative synthesis of findings. We assessed individual study quality using criteria based on the Newcastle-Ottawa quality assessment tools for observational studies. We assessed the overall strength of evidence for the body of included literature according to criteria developed by the GRADE Working Group.

A draft version of this report was reviewed by 11 technical experts, as well as clinical leadership. Reviewer comments were addressed and our responses were incorporated in the final report (Appendix G).

## RESULTS

From 2,668 titles and abstracts, we identified 354 articles for full-text review. Of these, 31 primary studies met inclusion criteria. In general, we found that though self-reported cognitive, physical, and mental health symptoms were common in the Veteran/military population, there was little evidence that symptoms were more common in those with mTBI than those without mTBI. However, the evidence base is weakened by inconsistent findings, methodologic shortcomings of many studies, and variation in outcomes considered and outcome measurement approaches. The following sections detail findings by symptom category.

### Summary of Cognitive Functioning Results

We found 17 studies reporting cognitive outcomes for those with mTBI. Overall, few studies found an association between mTBI and cognitive deficits. The strength of evidence is low overall because of poor and incomplete reporting of data and sampling procedures, lack of time-since-injury information, and because most studies were unblinded and single-center.

There were studies that found mTBI patients had deficits in visuospatial abilities, attention/concentration, and total/cross-domain composite scores as compared to patients without mTBI. However, even within each of these subdomains, findings were inconsistent across studies. In nearly all studies, scores for each of the subscales fell within normal limits, suggesting no clinically significant impairment in the group as a whole. Because studies did not report the proportion of patients scoring below normal range for each of the subscales, it is unclear whether there may have been subgroups of mTBI patients with cognitive deficits.

It is difficult to draw overall conclusions about which factors, in addition to mTBI, are independently associated with cognitive test performance since studies evaluated a variety of different factors and there were inconsistent findings among studies. Impaired cognitive test performance was associated with comorbid mental health diagnosis, time since injury of less than 10 days, self-reported cognitive complaints, and experiencing loss or alteration of consciousness at the time of injury.

# PREFACE

Quality Enhancement Research Initiative's (QUERI) Evidence-based Synthesis Program (ESP) was established to provide timely and accurate syntheses of targeted healthcare topics of particular importance to Veterans Affairs (VA) managers and policymakers, as they work to improve the health and healthcare of Veterans. The ESP disseminates these reports throughout VA.

QUERI provides funding for four ESP Centers and each Center has an active VA affiliation. The ESP Centers generate evidence syntheses on important clinical practice topics, and these reports help:

- develop clinical policies informed by evidence,
- guide the implementation of effective services to improve patient outcomes and to support VA clinical practice guidelines and performance measures, and
- set the direction for future research to address gaps in clinical knowledge.

In 2009, the ESP Coordinating Center was created to expand the capacity of QUERI Central Office and the four ESP sites by developing and maintaining program processes. In addition, the Center established a Steering Committee comprised of QUERI field-based investigators, VA Patient Care Services, Office of Quality and Performance, and Veterans Integrated Service Networks (VISN) Clinical Management Officers. The Steering Committee provides program oversight, guides strategic planning, coordinates dissemination activities, and develops collaborations with VA leadership to identify new ESP topics of importance to Veterans and the VA healthcare system.

Comments on this evidence report are welcome and can be sent to Nicole Floyd, ESP Coordinating Center Program Manager, at nicole.floyd@va.gov.

**Recommended citation:** O'Neil ME, Carlson KF, Storzbach D, Brenner LA, Freeman M, Quiñones A, Motu'apuaka M, Ensley M, Kansagara D. Complications of Mild Traumatic Brain Injury in Veterans and Military Personnel: A Systematic Review. VA-ESP Project #05-225; 2012

This report is based on research conducted by the Evidence-based Synthesis Program (ESP) Center located at the Portland VA Medical Center, Portland, OR funded by the Department of Veterans Affairs, Veterans Health Administration, Office of Research and Development, Quality Enhancement Research Initiative. The findings and conclusions in this document are those of the author(s) who are responsible for its contents; the findings and conclusions do not necessarily represent the views of the Department of Veterans Affairs or the United States government. Therefore, no statement in this article should be construed as an official position of the Department of Veterans Affairs. No investigators have any affiliations or financial involvement (e.g., employment, consultancies, honoraria, stock ownership or options, expert testimony, grants or patents received or pending, or royalties) that conflict with material presented in the report.

# TABLE OF CONTENTS

Self-reported cognitive complaints were common, both in Veterans with and without mTBI. Correlates of more severe self-reported cognitive problems include having an additional injury, loss of consciousness (LOC) or post-traumatic amnesia (PTA) at the time of injury versus only experiencing alteration of consciousness (AOC), being service connected, and having an Axis I mental health disorder.

## Summary of Physical Health Results

We found 17 studies reporting physical health outcomes for those with mTBI. Low strength evidence suggests that self-reported physical symptoms are associated with mTBI. This body of evidence is comprised entirely of low quality studies generally limited by poor and incomplete reporting of data and sampling procedures, by lack of time-since-injury information, and because most studies were unblinded and single-center.

Studies included in this report suggest that symptoms commonly reported by those with mTBI include headaches, pain, vestibular symptoms, hearing and vision problems, nausea or loss of appetite, and neurologic symptoms. One study reported that the prevalence of neurology referrals for headaches was 33.3% for Veterans with mTBI, though no other physical health studies reported prevalence estimates for these outcomes. It is also unclear whether mTBI directly contributes to the prevalence or severity of physical health symptoms as only two studies included a comparison group of participants without mTBI. Symptom severity ranged widely across individuals and many of the physical health outcomes were based solely on responses to an individual item from the Neurobehavioral Symptom Inventory (NSI), a general post-concussive symptom inventory. Additionally, inconsistent information on risk and protective factors provided insufficient evidence to make strong conclusions about potentially moderators of physical health outcomes.

## Summary of Mental Health Results

Twenty studies reported mental health outcomes for Veterans or members of the military with mTBI. Mental health outcomes varied greatly in terms of methods of assessment, ranging from lengthy clinical interviews based on diagnostic criteria, to single-item, self-report screeners. Overall, this body of literature provides low strength evidence, as it is based on low quality studies with many methodological limitations.

Studies included in this review suggest that there are high rates of mental health disorders and symptoms reported by Veterans and members of the military who have a history of mTBI. Prevalence of Axis I mental health disorders ranged from 50-78% in two studies; single studies reported that the rate of PTSD was 45%, alcohol abuse/dependence was 28%, drug abuse/dependence was 9%, suicidal ideation was 25%, suicidal intent was 7%, and past suicide attempts was 4% for Veterans with mTBI. Notably, however, the majority of included studies suggest that there are few, if any, significant differences in mental health outcomes for those with mTBI compared to Veteran/military participants without mTBI. Finally, though many individual studies investigated potential moderating factors for mental health outcomes, no clear risk or protective factors were identified.

## Summary of Functional/Social Outcome Results

We found 12 studies, all low quality, reporting functional/social outcomes for Veterans or members of the military with mTBI. Due to methodologic limitations as well as small sample size and inadequate reporting of and accounting for time since injury, the strength of evidence for this group of studies is low. One study reported that approximately 20% of Veterans with mTBI experience unemployment. One of two studies comparing participants with and without mTBI found higher unemployment among those with mTBI. Another study found that 26% of those with mTBI had difficulties with interpersonal relationships, though this was not significantly different in comparison to individuals without mTBI. Ten studies examined sleep disturbance: two found an overall prevalence of 13-23%, and seven found that sleep disturbances, when present, were moderate to severe. One of two studies found that sleep disturbance was more common in those with mTBI compared to those without. No clear patterns of risk or protective factors emerged from studies examining potential moderators of associations between mTBI and functional or social outcomes.

## Summary of Service Utilization/Cost Results

We found seven low quality studies that described service utilization by those with mTBI, but no studies that reported costs associated with mTBI. The overall strength of evidence was low because of the small number and methodologic shortcomings of studies. The available literature suggests that there are few differences in service utilization for those with mTBI compared to similar controls; no significant associations with risk or protective factors were identified.

## Conclusion

Overall, given the low strength of evidence, it is difficult to draw firm conclusions about the effects of mTBI in Veteran and military populations. The literature reviewed here is relatively consistent with findings from the more methodologically rigorous, prospective, longitudinal studies conducted in civilian populations. Both bodies of literature suggest that though some negative outcomes occur for a significant portion of individuals who have mTBI, most objective results (e.g., objective cognitive test results) are not significantly different from control participants, and deficits that are present shortly following injury most often resolve within days to months. The literature on Veterans and members of the military suggests that many have physical and mental health symptoms, but it is not clear that those with mTBI experience more or higher severity symptoms than those without mTBI suggesting that outcomes may be influenced by other deployment-related conditions such as PTSD. The studies included in this report were low quality, cross sectional studies which did not provide consistent evidence for potential moderators of mTBI outcomes.

# LIMITATIONS AND FUTURE RESEARCH

One of the major limitations of this literature is the inadequate reporting of and accounting for time since injury. Future research on Veterans and members of the military should not only report time since injury for their research populations, but specifically account for time since injury in their analyses so that outcomes can be analyzed over time.

Few studies presented data on all outcomes of interest to the stakeholders of this review, and few studies reported their outcome reporting rationale. Most studies relied on clinical datasets, rather than research databases or registries. It is likely that many studies only included outcomes of relevance to the authors' particular study questions, though it is impossible to know whether some studies did not report outcomes given a lack of association with mTBI. There is a pressing need for large cohort studies of Veterans with and without mTBI that prospectively collect data on all risk and protective factors, and all outcomes of interest. Such studies would be relatively costly but would result in higher-quality evidence on which more definitive conclusions could be based.

Very few studies reported the actual prevalence of symptoms or conditions; most studies simply reported mean scores for the entire study group. Future research should report proportions of individuals with clinically significant impairment for each outcome.

Although a strength of this review was that many of the included studies relied on well-validated measures commonly used with Veteran/military populations, many of the clinical outcomes relied solely on self-reported symptoms, often obtained from single items on questionnaires. Results from this review and from the civilian literature suggest that self-reported deficits are more likely to be reported by individuals with mTBI compared to similar individuals without mTBI, particularly when associated with potential financial compensation. Future research should use objective and validated assessments, blinded outcome assessors, patient blinding to study hypotheses, and accounting for compensation factors whenever possible in order to reduce potential bias associated with outcome assessment. Additionally, future research should employ commonly used outcome assessment tools in order to facilitate the combination of results across studies for meta-analytic purposes.

A final strength of this review was the use of clear criteria for defining mTBI, as established by the VA and DoD. However, because the majority of studies did not assess or report imaging results, a key component of the VA/DoD criteria for mTBI, we were unable to use positive imaging results as an exclusion criteria. Future primary research should clearly report criteria used to define mTBI, including assessment and reporting of imaging results when available, and should consider examination of differences in outcomes based on definitional criteria for mTBI, as it is possible that less stringent criteria could be associated with different results.

## ABBREVIATIONS TABLE

| | |
|---|---|
| ACRM | American Congress of Rehabilitation Medicine |
| AFB | Air Force Base |
| AIS | Abbreviated Injury Scale |
| AMC | Army Medical Center |
| ANAM | Automated Neuropsychological Assessment Metrics |
| AOC | Alteration of Consciousness/Mental State |
| BAMC | Brooke Army Medical Center |
| BDI-II | Beck Depression Inventory 2nd Edition |
| BTBIS | Brief Traumatic Brain Injury Screen |
| BVMT-R | Brief Visuospatial Memory Test Revised |
| C&P | Compensation and Pension |
| CAPS | Clinician Administered PTSD Scale |

| | |
|---|---|
| CDC | Centers for Disease Control and Prevention |
| CDD | ANAM - code substitution delayed |
| CDS | ANAM - code substitution |
| CI | Confidence Interval |
| COWA | Controlled Oral Word Association |
| CT | Computed tomography |
| CTE | Chronic Traumatic Encephalopathy |
| CVAMC | Cleveland Veterans Affairs Medical Center |
| CVLT-II | California Verbal Learning Test Second Edition |
| DHI | Dizziness Handicap Inventory |
| D-KEFS | Delis-Kaplan Executive Function System Trail Making subtests |
| DoD | Department of Defense |
| DTI | Diffusion Tensor Imaging |
| DVBIC | Defense and Veterans Brain Injury Center |
| DVAT | Dynamic Visual Acuity Test |
| EFP | Explosively Formed Projectile |
| ESS | Epworth Sleepiness Scale |
| FCES | Full Combat Exposure Scale |
| FrSBe | Frontal Systems Behavioral Scale |
| FSIQ | Estimated Full Scale IQ |
| GED | General Educational Development |
| GCS | Glasgow Coma Scale |
| HADS | Hospital Anxiety and Depression Scale |
| HIT-6 | Headache Impact Test-6 |
| HS | High School |
| ICU | Average days in ICU |
| IED | Improvised explosive device |
| IQR | Interquartile range |
| ISS | Injury Severity Scale |
| LOC | Loss of consciousness |
| LOS | Length of stay |
| MACE | Military Acute Concussion Evaluation |
| mBIAS | Mild brain injury atypical symptoms scale |
| MIDAS | Migraine Disability Assessment Score |
| MIRECC | Mental Illness Research, Education and Clinical Center |
| MOCA | Montreal Cognitive Assessment |
| MRI | Magnetic Resonance Imaging |
| MSP | ANAM - matching to sample |
| mTBI | Mild traumatic brain injury |
| MTH | ANAM - mathematical processing |
| MVA | Motor vehicle accident |
| NA | Not applicable |
| NR | Not Reported |
| NSI | Neurobehavioral Symptom Inventory |
| OEF | Operation Enduring Freedom |
| OIF | Operation Iraqi Freedom |

| | |
|---|---|
| OND | Operation New Dawn |
| OR | Odds Ratio |
| PCL | PTSD Checklist |
| PCL-C | PTSD Checklist, Civilian version |
| PCL-M | PTSD Checklist, Military version |
| PCL-S | PTSD Checklist Stressor Specific Version |
| PCS | Postconcussive symptoms |
| PHQ-15 | Patient Health Questionnaire—15 |
| PI | Principal Investigator |
| PM&R | Physical Medicine and Rehabilitation |
| PRT | Procedural reaction time |
| PT | Physical training |
| PTA | Post-traumatic amnesia |
| PTSD | Posttraumatic Stress Disorder |
| RBANS | Repeatable Battery for the Assessment of Neuropsychological Status |
| RCFT | Rey Complex Figure Test |
| Rey FIT | Rey 15 Item test |
| ROCFT | Rey Osterlith Complex Figure Test |
| RPG | Rocket propelled grenade |
| SAC | Standardized assessment of concussion |
| SCID-I | Structured Clinical Interview for DSM-IV Axis I Disorders |
| SD | Standard deviation |
| SR | Systematic review |
| SRT | Simple reaction time |
| TBI | Traumatic brain injury |
| TOMM | Test of Memory Malingering |
| VACO | Veterans Affairs Central Office |
| VAMC | Veterans Affairs Medical Center |
| VBIED | Vehicle borne improvised explosive device |
| VHA | Veterans Health Administration |
| VISN | Veterans Integrated Service Network |
| VSVT | Victoria Symptom Validity Test |
| WAIS-III | Wechsler Adult Intelligence Scale Third Edition |
| WAIS-IV | Wechsler Adult Intelligence Scale Version IV |
| WASI | Wechsler Abbreviated Scale of Intelligence |
| WHO | World Health Organization |
| WMS-III | Wechsler Memory Scale Third Edition |
| WRAMC | Walter Reed Army Medical Center |
| WTAR | Wechsler Test of Adult Reading |

# EVIDENCE REPORT

## INTRODUCTION

Traumatic brain injury (TBI) is a common condition, especially among military members. Twelve to 23 percent of service members returning from Operations Enduring Freedom, Iraqi Freedom, and New Dawn (OEF/OIF/OND) experienced a TBI while deployed. Although various criteria are used to define TBI severity, the majority of documented TBI events among OEF/OIF/OND service members may be classified as mild in severity, or mTBI, according to the definition used by the Veterans Health Administration and Department of Defense (VA/DoD).[1]

While some researchers suggest most individuals recover within three months of an mTBI, others estimate that 10 to 20 percent of individuals continue to experience post-concussive symptoms (e.g., headaches, dizziness, balance problems) beyond this time fame.[2] This estimate may be higher among OEF/OIF service members given the frequency of multiple TBI events, concomitant mental health conditions such as depression and posttraumatic stress disorder (PTSD), and other factors unique to combat deployments. As such, deployment-related mTBI is a significant issue for the VA, as patients who report ongoing mTBI symptoms may require the attention from a range of health care professionals.[3] This evidence synthesis review will be used by the VHA TBI Advisory Committee to develop strategies to identify those at-risk for long-term mTBI effects, inform clinical practice, determine resource allocation, and identify future research priorities.

# METHODS

## TOPIC DEVELOPMENT

This project was nominated by Dr. Stuart Hoffman, Scientific Program Manager for the Brain Injury portfolio, Rehabilitation Research & Development Service. Operational partners include David X. Cifu, MD, Chair, VHA TBI Advisory Committee and National Director of Physical Medicine and Rehabilitation (PM&R) Program Office; Robert L. Ruff, MD, PhD, National Director for Neurology and Acting-Director of Rehabilitation Research and Development; Joel Scholten, MD, Associate Chief of Staff for Rehabilitation Services, Washington DC VA Medical Center Director of Special Projects, PM&R Program Office, Veterans Affairs Central Office (VACO); and Alexander Ommaya, DSc, Director of Translational Research, Office of Research and Development. We also received input from a technical expert panel.

Anticipated report usage:

The evidence synthesis review will be used by the VHA TBI Advisory Committee to develop strategies to determine which sub-groups are most at risk for long-term effects of mTBI. The review will be used to inform clinical practice and to identify how best to allocate future resources for effective screening for late complications of mTBI. The review will also identify gaps in evidence that warrant further research.

The final key questions are:

Key Question #1. For Veteran/military populations, what is the prevalence of health problems (such as pain, seizure disorders, headaches, migraines, and vertigo), cognitive deficits, functional limitations (such as employment status, changes in marital status/family dynamics), and mental health symptoms (such as PTSD and depression) that develop or persist following mTBI?

Key Question #2. What factors affect outcomes for Veteran/military patients with mTBI? Key Question 2A: For Veteran/military populations, are there pre-injury (premorbid) risk/protective factors (e.g., pre-injury mental health factors, genetic factors, or prior concussions) that affect outcomes for mTBI? Key Question 2B: For Veteran/military populations, are there post-injury risk/protective factors (e.g., PTSD) that affect outcomes for mTBI?

Key Question #3. What is the resource utilization over time for Veteran/military patients with mTBI?

## SEARCH STRATEGY

We searched Medline, PsychINFO and Cochrane Register of Controlled Trials (OVID) for observational studies, clinical trials, systematic reviews, and cost studies, from database inception to October 3rd, 2012. We limited the search to articles involving human subjects and published in the English language. We adapted the search strategy developed by the WHO Collaborating Centre for Neurotrauma Prevention, Management and Rehabilitation Task Force for a recent systematic review of prognosis after mTBI, which included the terms 'traumatic brain injury,' 'craniocerebral trauma,' 'prognosis,' and 'recovery of function.'[4] The full details of the search strategy are provided in Appendix A. The preliminary WHO Collaborating Centre for Neurotrauma Prevention, Management and Rehabilitation Task Force search strategy was reviewed by a library scientist and by our team of investigators with clinical expertise in order to assure comprehensiveness of the search. The search was expanded to include additional mTBI search terminology following the discovery of a relevant article which was not identified in the preliminary search. After review, we expanded the WHO Collaborating Centre for Neurotrauma Prevention, Management and Rehabilitation Task Force search with additional TBI terms and also limited the search to Veteran/military population studies by using terms including military, VA, and Veteran (Appendix A). We obtained additional articles from systematic reviews, reference lists of pertinent studies, reviews, editorials, and by consulting clinical and research experts. All citations were imported into an electronic database (EndNote X4).

## STUDY SELECTION

We included studies reporting outcomes in Veterans or military personnel who had suffered an mTBI using a case definition consistent with definitions in the VA/DoD Clinical Practice Guideline for Management of Concussion/Mild Traumatic Brain Injury. Abstracts of citations identified from literature searches were reviewed by the PI to assess for relevance to the key questions; a portion of the abstracts were dual reviewed by at least one additional member of the team to assure accuracy and consistency of coding. Full-text articles of potentially relevant abstracts were retrieved for further review, and reviewed by the PI and at least one additional reviewer. Full-text articles for which there was disagreement by two reviewers were reviewed by the team of investigators and included or excluded based on team consensus. Each article was reviewed using the eligibility criteria in Appendix B. A list of excluded studies grouped by reason for exclusion is reported in Appendix F. Eligible articles had English-language abstracts and provided data relevant to the key questions. Articles also had to report outcomes for members of the U.S. armed forces or Veterans.

Diagnostically, to have sustained a TBI one must have experienced an event (e.g., motor vehicle crash, fall) which resulted in a structural injury to the brain or a physiological disruption of brain function (e.g., alteration of consciousness,[5] loss of consciousness [LOC], or post-traumatic amnesia[6]). TBI severity is classified according to the extent of harm to the brain or altered consciousness associated with the injury. Severity of residual symptoms reported or observed should not be used to classify TBI severity. Therefore, to apply consistent criteria to define mTBI and compare similar populations with mTBI, all included studies had to use a definition of mTBI consistent with the VA/Department of Defense (DoD) Clinical Practice Guideline for Management of Concussion/Mild Traumatic Brain Injury described in Appendix C. Articles that described their populations as having mTBI but used definitions of mTBI differing from the VA/DoD criteria were excluded from this evidence synthesis but are described in Appendix D. Due to the frequent lack of reporting or obtaining imaging results (e.g., MRI, CT scan), the only variation from this definition in included studies relates to positive imaging results: we included studies regardless of whether they reported or included participants with positive imaging results as long as the rest of their mTBI inclusion criteria were consistent with the VA/DoD criteria. Finally, we did not limit study eligibility based on number of mTBI incidents or the presence of comorbid conditions.

We published our key questions and abstract online so that they were available for public review. A summary of article inclusion criteria is as follows:

Population(s): Veterans or members of the military who have experienced mTBI. Studies that do not differentiate between adult and child populations, or between Veteran/military and civilian populations, will be excluded. Studies must state a clear case definition for mTBI that falls within the definitions provided by the VA/DoD Clinical Practice Guideline for Management of Concussion/Mild Traumatic Brain Injury (Appendix C).

Intervention(s): Not applicable to the proposed key questions.

Comparator(s): Similar populations that have not been diagnosed with mTBI or concussion; comparison group not required for inclusion.

Outcome(s): Health problems (e.g., pain, seizure disorders, chronic headaches, migraines, vertigo, etc.), cognitive deficits, functional limitations (e.g., employment status, marital status changes/family dynamic changes), mental health symptoms (e.g., diagnosis of PTSD or depression), and cost/resource utilization (ER visits, hospitalizations, outpatient appointments). Outcomes diagnosed post-mortem will be included (e.g., Chronic Traumatic Encephalopathy [CTE]).

Timing: No limitations based on time since injury.

Setting: No limitations based on study setting.

Study design: Systematic reviews, meta-analyses, randomized controlled trials, prospective and retrospective cohort studies, case control studies, case series, and cross-sectional studies.

Sample size: All included studies must include a minimum of 30 mTBI cases, so that a better level of precision and confidence in the results can be achieved.

## DATA ABSTRACTION

We abstracted the following data for each included study: sample selection, population characteristics, subject eligibility and exclusion criteria, number of subjects, comparison(s), and outcome(s) (See Table 1 and Appendix E). Data was abstracted by one investigator and reviewed for accuracy by at least one additional investigator.

## QUALITY ASSESSMENT

We assessed the quality of included studies pertaining to all of the key questions. We found no randomized trials meeting inclusion criteria, and our entire sample of included studies is comprised of observational studies of various designs, primarily retrospective cohort, case control, and case series. Issues of quality, particularly in observational studies, are often unique to the condition and outcomes of interest. Therefore, though we assessed quality using criteria based on the Newcastle-Ottawa quality assessment tools for observational studies[7] the criteria that specifically related to this body of literature included the following: accurate definition of condition of interest, consecutive sample selection, use of validated assessment tools, blinding of outcome assessors, blinding of patients and assessors to study hypotheses, adjustment for known confounders including mental health condition, comparability of controls, response rate, attrition, and reduced risk of reporting bias. These indicators of study quality and potential for bias were abstracted by one investigator and reviewed for accuracy by at least one additional investigator who was not blinded to the original assessment. In cases of disagreement, the team of investigators reviewed the study and came to consensus on quality assessment. In addition to quality rating of individual studies, we evaluated the overall quality of the evidence for each key question as proposed by the GRADE Working Group.[8]

## DATA SYNTHESIS

We constructed evidence tables showing the study characteristics and results for all included studies organized by outcome. We critically analyzed studies to compare their characteristics, methods, and findings. We compiled a summary of findings for each outcome category and key question, and drew conclusions based on qualitative synthesis of the findings. We did not combine the studies in a quantitative manner via meta-analysis because of the heterogeneity of outcomes and study characteristics. The synthesis was conducted by the principal investigator, though all results were reviewed with the team of investigators to review and obtain consensus on the reported findings.

## RATING THE BODY OF EVIDENCE

We assessed the overall quality of evidence for outcomes using a method developed by the GRADE Working Group,[8] which classified the grade of evidence across outcomes according to the following criteria:

- High = Further research is very unlikely to change our confidence on the estimate of effect.
- Moderate = Further research is likely to have an important impact on our confidence in the estimate of effect and may change the estimate.
- Low = Further research is very likely to have an important impact on our confidence in the estimate of effect and is likely to change the estimate.
- Very Low = Any estimate of effect is very uncertain.

## PEER REVIEW

A draft version of this report was reviewed by 11 technical experts as well as clinical leadership. Their comments and our responses are presented in Appendix G.

# RESULTS

## METHODOLOGIC CONSIDERATIONS

The strengths of included studies include using well-validated assessment tools, comparing similar populations with and without mTBI, and applying a clearly reported definition of mTBI consistent with VA/DoD criteria. In spite of these strengths, however, all of the included studies were rated as having high risk of bias for the following reasons: The included studies often did not adequately account for time since injury (the only exception being two studies reporting results from a single population), or other quality factors such as assessor blinding to the presence of mTBI, participant and assessor blinding to study hypotheses, or clearly reporting sampling procedures. This body of observational literature did not, in general, report results in a manner consistent with reduced reporting bias, and it is possible that studies emphasized or only reported statistically significant or otherwise selected results. Because outcomes and risk/ protective factors are often described in single studies without replication by other research teams, this body of literature is not strengthened by adequate replication and confirmation of preliminary results. Therefore, the overall body of literature providing evidence on outcomes for those with mTBI is from low quality observational studies, and the overall strength of evidence is low for all outcomes reported in this review. Because all individual studies were rated as having high risk of bias, no studies were differentially weighted based on quality in the data synthesis.

## LITERATURE FLOW

We reviewed 2,664 titles and abstracts from the electronic search, and identified an additional 4 studies from reviewing reference lists and conducting manual searches. After applying inclusion/ exclusion criteria at the abstract level, 354 full-text articles were reviewed, as shown in Figure 1. Of the full-text articles, we excluded 323 that did not meet inclusion criteria. We grouped the studies by outcome and key question. Figure 1 details the exclusion criteria and the number of references related to each of the key questions. We identified 31 primary studies that addressed the key questions. All studies were conducted in U.S. Veterans or active-duty service members of the U.S. military. Table 1 shows the characteristics of the 31 primary studies, and the following sections detail findings according to symptom category.

**Figure 1. Literature Flow Diagram**

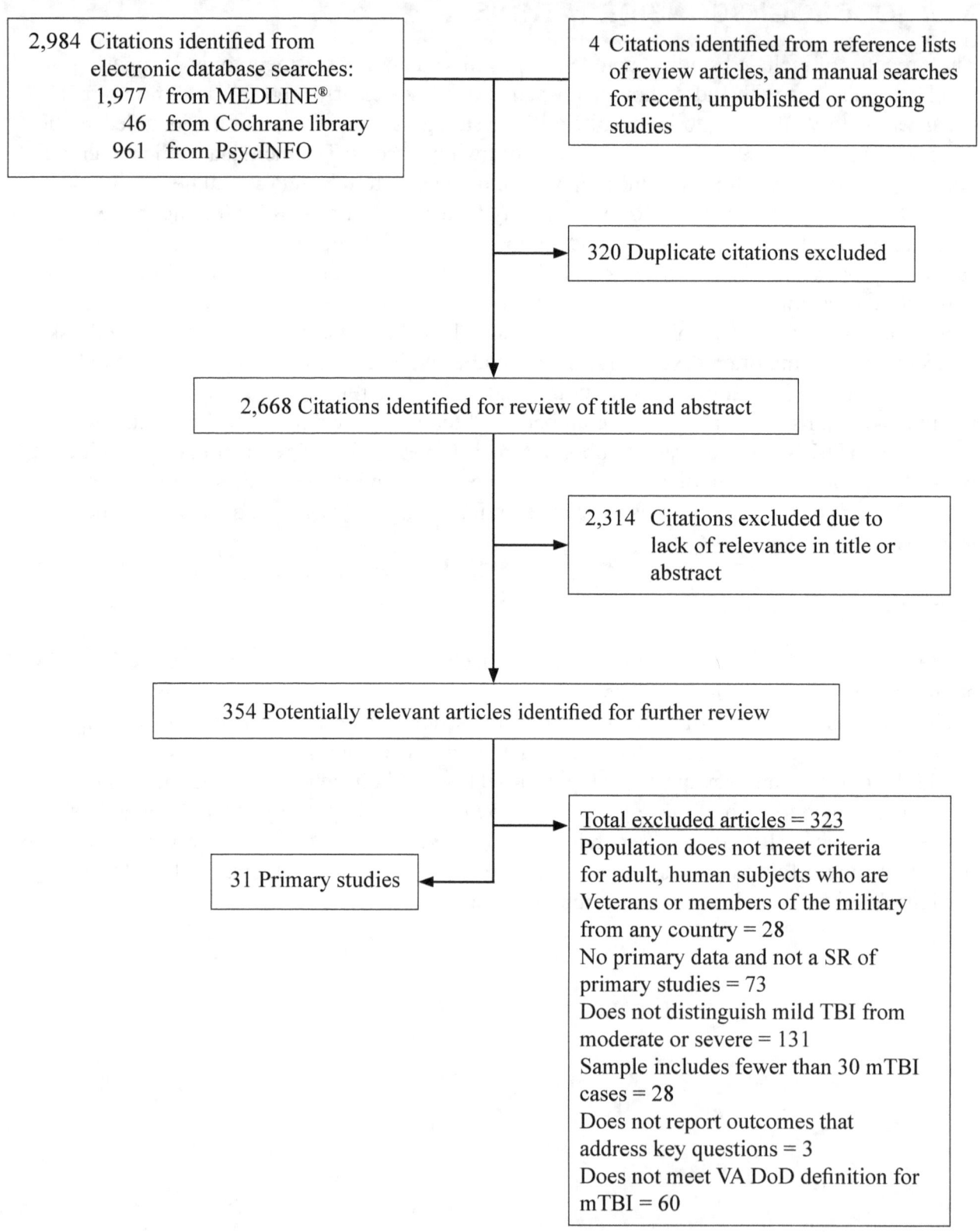

**Table 1. Descriptive Characteristics of Studies of U.S. Veterans and Members of the U.S. Military with Mild Traumatic Brain Injury**

| Author, year | Population and sample selection | Sample size: Total, mTBI | mTBI definition and associated citation reported in the study | Demographics of mTBI group | Time since injury for mTBI group, Mean (SD); Mechanism of injury; Prior TBI |
|---|---|---|---|---|---|
| Barnes, Walter, & Chard, 2012[9] | Consecutive referrals for outpatient PTSD treatment between 2006 and 2010 at a Midwestern Veterans Affairs Medical Center. All patients served in OEF and/ or OIF and met diagnostic criteria for PTSD due to combat-related trauma. Excluded: LOC >30 mins or PTA >24 hrs. | 92, 46 | • Definition: AOC, LOC, PTA. <br>• Positive imaging: NR <br>• Citation: Holm, Cassidy, Carroll, & Borg, 2005 <br>• How assessed: Chart review, clinical interview | (data reported only for entire sample) <br>• Age: 30.3 (8.2) <br>• Gender: 100% male <br>• Race/Ethnicity: 93.3% Caucasian, 4.4% African American, 2.2% Native American <br>• Education: NR | • Time since injury: NR <br>• Mechanism of Injury: NR <br>• Prior TBI: NR |
| Belanger, Kretzmer, Vanderploeg, & French, 2010[10] | Patients consecutively admitted to Tampa VAMC or WRAMC; clinics not specified. | 225, 134 | • Definition: PTA, LOC <br>• Positive Imaging: Excluded <br>• Citation: Kay et al., 1993 <br>• How assessed: Self report, chart review | • Age: 30.7 (9.5) <br>• Gender: 97% male <br>• Race/Ethnicity: NR <br>• Education: NR | • Time since injury: 703.5 (1064.1) days <br>• Mechanism of Injury: 67% blast, 25% MVA, 7% other mechanism of injury <br>• Prior TBI: 14/134 with prior mTBI |
| Belanger, Kretzmer, Yoash-Gantz, Pickett, & Tupler, 2009[11] | Tampa and Richmond VA consecutive brain injury rehab patients referred for neuropsychological evaluation; Salisbury and Durham VAMC post-deployment and VA outpatients; and "selected research volunteers" from Mid-Atlantic MIRECC. Excluded: poor effort or malingering based on clinical presentation and/or if they failed certain measures of symptom validity; neurological disorders; brain injury due to gunshot. | 102, 51 | • Definition: LOC and PTA <br>• Positive Imaging: Included (n = 6 blast, n = 3 non-blast) <br>• Citation: Kay et al., 1993 <br>• How assessed: Self-report, chart review | • Age: 30.9 (9.2) <br>• Gender: NR* (4/102 female for entire aggregate sample) <br>• Race/Ethnicity: NR* (76 Caucasian, 16 African American; 8 Hispanic; 2 Other for entire aggregate sample) <br>• Education: 13.1 (2.2) yrs | • Time since injury: 1021.4 (1730.0) days <br>• Mechanism of Injury: For total sample: 49 = blast only; 12 = blast plus MVA, 41 = non-blast <br>• Prior TBI: NR* (n = 20 for entire aggregate sample) |
| Belanger, Proctor-Weber, Kretzmer, et al. 2011[12] | Tampa and Bay Pines VAMCs and WRAMC. 10% of these participants were included in the Belanger, Kretzmer, Vanderploeg, & French, 2010 analyses. | 390 | • Definition: DoD Criteria <br>• Positive Imaging: Excluded <br>• Citation: Kay et al., 1993 <br>• How assessed: Clinical interview chart review | • Age: 28.3 (7.9) for blast exposed; 30.0 (9.1) for non-blast exposed <br>• Gender: 94% male <br>• Race/Ethnicity: NR <br>• Education: NR | • Time since injury: 6 months (WRAMC); 52 months (VA) <br>• Mechanism of Injury: 298 = blast, 92 = non-blast cause <br>• Prior TBI: NR |
| Benge, Pastorek, & Thornton, 2009[13] | Veterans evaluated by the polytrauma team. Excluded: moderate or severe brain injury; skull penetration. | 345 | • Definition: Identifying a mechanism of injury and endorsing at least one of the following symptoms: LOC, PTA, or feeling dazed for <24 hrs after the injury. <br>• Positive imaging: NR <br>• Citation: Defense and Veterans Brain Injury Center, 2006 <br>• How assessed: Chart review | • Age: 30.4 (7.5) <br>• Gender: 96.2% male <br>• Race/Ethnicity: 11.6% African American, 66.4% White, 18.6% Hispanic, 3.5% other <br>• Education: 55.9% HS diploma or equivalent, 37.1% some college, 5.8% college graduate, 1.2% other | • Time since injury: 3.0 (1.6) yrs (most recent injury) <br>• Mechanism of Injury: 64.6% report at least one blast injury, 29.9 report at least one motor vehicle accident, 25.5 report at least one fall <br>• Prior TBI: NR |

| Author, year | Population and sample selection | mTBI definition and associated citation reported in the study | Sample size: Total, mTBI | Demographics of mTBI group | Time since injury for mTBI group, Mean (SD); Mechanism of injury; Prior TBI |
|---|---|---|---|---|---|
| Coldren, Kelly, Parish, et al., 2010[14] | Jan 11, 2009-Apr 10, 2009, U.S. Army soldiers presenting for medical care within 72 hrs of suffering a concussive event in Iraq. Included: 18-50 years, meeting DoD definition of a concussion, free of psychoactive medication, no significant psychiatric diagnosis requiring ongoing therapy, reporting pain not greater than 7 on a scale of I to 10, consenting to be in the study. Subjects and controls were enrolled from Victory Base Complex, Joint Base Balad, and Mosul. Non-TBI injured controls were patients in the same timeframe. Healthy controls were volunteers located at same base. Excluded: any history of severe TBI, moderate TBI within the previous 3 yrs, or of any concussion within 90 days of current injury. | • Definition: DoD criteria <br> • Positive imaging: NR <br> • Citation: DoD diagnostic criteria, no citation given <br> • How assessed: Clinical interview | 237, 71 | Cases vs. controls: <br> • Age: 26.5 vs. 27.3 (SD not reported), p = 0.44 <br> • Gender: 96% vs. 88% male, p = 0.07 <br> • Race/Ethnicity: NR <br> • Education (yrs): 12.5 vs. 13.1 (SD not reported), p = 0.02 | • Time since injury: within 72 hrs <br> • Mechanism of Injury: NR <br> • Prior TBI: Excluded moderate or severe TBI within 3 yrs, and concussion within 90 days of current injury. |
| Coldren, Russell, Parish, et al., 2012[15] | US Army soldiers presenting to an outpatient medical facility within 72 hrs of a concussion between January to April, 2009; free of cognition altering medication or severe psychiatric diagnosis requiring ongoing therapy, no pain > 7 on a 1-10 scale, no severe TBI, no moderate TBI within the past 3 yrs, no concussion within the past 90 days. | • Definition: DoD criteria <br> • Positive imaging: NR <br> • Citation: NR <br> • How assessed: NR | 235, 69 | • Age: 18-20 (9%), 21-25 (45%), 26-30 (26%), 31-40 (17%), 41-55( 4%) <br> • Gender: 96% male <br> • Race/Ethnicity: Caucasian (72%), Black (4%), Hispanic (19%), other (4%) <br> • Education: HS (4%), HS graduate (57%), some college (38%), college graduate (0%) | • Time since injury: 0 (2%), 1 (47%), 2 (29%), 3 (22%) days <br> • Mechanism of Injury: blast 45%, blow 26%, mixed 11%, unknown 19% <br> • Prior TBI: none in past 90 days |
| Cooper, Chau, Armistead-Jehle et al., 2012[16] | Consecutive admissions of OEF/OIF military service members referred to the TBI clinic at BAMC for neuropsychological testing between January 2008 and January 2010. All participants were over 18 years of age, spoke English fluently, and were injured while on active duty. Excluded participants had major body burns, had traumatic amputations, were missing key variable data, or performed below cutoffs indicating suboptimal effort on neuropsychological measures. No psychiatric exclusion criteria were applied. | • Definition: ACRM and VA/DoD criteria <br> • Positive imaging: Excluded <br> • Citation: ACRM, 1993 <br> • How assessed: Clinical interview and chart review | 60 | Blast exposed vs. non-blast exposed: <br> • Age: 29.5 (7.73) vs. 29.43 (7.95) <br> • Gender: 100% vs. 78.6% male <br> • Race/Ethnicity: NR <br> • Education: NR | Blast exposed vs. non-blast exposed: <br> • Time since injury: 192.29 (167.46), 148.69 (150.98) days <br> • Mechanism of Injury: Blast 53% non-blast 47% <br> • Prior TBI: NR |

| Author, year | Population and sample selection | mTBI definition and associated citation reported in the study | Sample size: Total, mTBI | Demographics of mTBI group | Time since injury for mTBI group, Mean (SD); Mechanism of injury; Prior TBI |
|---|---|---|---|---|---|
| Cooper, Kennedy, Cullen, et al., 2011[17] | Active duty service members, including activated reservists and members of the National Guard, who were evaluated at a military medical treatment facility in Brooke Army Medical Center (BAMC) following a combat deployment to Iraq or Afghanistan and sustained a concussive injury during their deployment. Subjects were identified for this study through multiple sources including inpatient care, post-deployment primary care clinics, specialty care clinics (e.g. Traumatic Brain Injury Service) and case management. Excluded: did not sustain a TBI, 87 subjects with moderate or severe TBI or penetrating brain injuries; 232 mTBI subjects with PCL-C scores 31–59 from this analysis to maximize the dispersion of the combat stress variable (i.e., excluded medium-combat stress in order to compare low vs. high). | • Definition: ACRM criteria.<br>• Positive imaging: NR<br>• Citation: ACRM, 1993<br>• How assessed: Clinical interview | 240 | Low combat stress vs. high combat stress:<br>• Age: 26.4 (6.5) vs. 27.8 (6.9)<br>• Gender: 99.2% vs. 94.4%<br>• Race/Ethnicity: NR<br>• Education: NR | Low combat stress vs. high combat stress:<br>• Time since injury: 3.8 (5.8) vs. 7.3 (11.0) months<br>• Mechanism of Injury: Blast 84% vs. 85%<br>• Prior TBI: NR |
| Cooper, Mercado-Couch, Richfield, et al, 2010[18] | 194 US military service members with burn injuries due to explosive munitions treated at BAMC between Sep 2005 and Oct 2007. Service members who sustained a blast injury were referred to the Neuropsychology Service as part of routine screening for clinical evaluation and neurocognitive testing. Excluded: 10 participants due to length of PTA suggesting a more severe brain injury than ACRM criteria; 17 subjects because they could not complete the manual portion of neuropsychological testing due to severe bilateral burns and/or amputations. | • Definition: ACRM criteria; and GCS score ≥ 13<br>• Positive imaging: NR<br>• Citation: ACRM, 1993<br>• How assessed: Clinical interview and chart review | 167, 50 | TBI+ (n = 50) vs. TBI- (n = 117):<br>• Age: 25.06 (5.818) vs. 25.67 (5.537), p = 0.524<br>• Gender: 44 (88.0%) male 114 vs. (97.4%) male, p = 0.013<br>• Race/Ethnicity: NR<br>• Education (presumably years): 12.54 (1.073) vs. 12.52 (1.454), p = 0.935 | TBI+ vs. TBI-<br>• Weeks since injury: 8.12 (7.763) vs. 7.76 (8.181), p = 0.792<br>• Mechanism of Injury: All subjects had burn injuries due to explosive munitions<br>• Prior TBI: NR |
| Cooper, Nelson, Armistead-Jehle, et al., 2011[19] | Consecutive referrals to a Brain Injury clinic, including documented or suspected mTBI and neurorehabilitation patients. The sample was primarily composed of active duty service members including activated reservists and members of the National Guard. As part of standard operating procedure, all individuals referred to the clinic completed self- report symptom questionnaires on a computer kiosk prior to their initial encounter with a medical provider. Only subjects completing all three self-report questionnaires. (PCL-M; NSI; mBIAS) were included in the final sample. From an initial archival set of 443 subjects, 40 subjects were excluded for incomplete data on one or more measures of interest. | • Definition: ACRM criteria; GCS score ≥ 13. Consistent with the current DoD guidance ... individuals with positive neuroimaging findings, who otherwise met criteria for mTBI, were classified as moderate TBI.<br>• Positive imaging: Excluded<br>• Citation: Casscells, 2007; ACRM, 2003<br>• How assessed: Clinical interview, chart review | 403, 268 | • Age: 32 (9)<br>• Gender: 93% male<br>• Race/Ethnicity: NR<br>• Education: NR | • Time since injury: N (%)<br>1 yr: N = 148 (62%)<br>1-3 yrs: N = 53 (22%)<br>>3 yrs: N = 35 (15%)<br>• Mechanism of Injury: NR<br>• Prior TBI: NR |

| Author, year | Population and sample selection | mTBI definition and associated citation reported in the study | Sample size; Total, mTBI | Demographics of mTBI group | Time since injury for mTBI group, Mean (SD); Mechanism of injury; Prior TBI |
|---|---|---|---|---|---|
| Drag, Spencer, Walker, et al., 2012[20] | Veterans in TBI clinic at the VA Ann Arbor Healthcare System, consecutive sample. Excluded injuries exceeding a mTBI; C and P evaluation; scored below cutoff on Digit Span; scored below cutoff on the Rey-15; incomplete data; scored below cutoff on the Shipley Vocabulary test. | • Definition: LOC; PTA; "alteration in mental state" at time of injury; focal neurological deficit <br> • Positive imaging: NR <br> • Citation: Kay et al., 1993 <br> • How assessed: Self-report screening tool and structured clinical interview | 167 | • Age: 29.47 (7.28) <br> • Gender: 163 (M), 4 (F) <br> • Race/Ethnicity: NR <br> • Education: 12.89 (1.63) yrs | • Time since injury: 41.93 (34.06) months <br> • Mechanism of Injury: NR <br> • Prior TBI: NR |
| Gaylord, Cooper, Mercado, et al., 2008[21] | The population at risk included 360 service members admitted to the USAISR Burn Center for burn and explosion injuries from Aug 2004 to Aug 2006. 146 burned service members treated at the USAISR Burn Center were assessed for PTSD during Sep 2005 through Aug 2006. Of these, 80 were also assessed for TBI. Subjects were included in the study if they sustained both a burn and blast injury and were assessed for both PTSD and TBI (n = 80). Two subjects were diagnosed for moderate and severe TBI and were excluded. Two subjects were excluded because they were not injured in OEF or OIF. Subjects with moderate or severe TBI (as defined by GCS <12 and duration of PTA >24 hrs) were excluded from the current study. | • Definition: ACRM criteria; and a GCS score ≥ 13. <br> • Positive imaging: NR <br> • Citation: ACRM, 1993 <br> • How assessed: Clinical interview | 76, 31 | • Age: 25.5. (6) mTBI plus PTSD 25, mTBI no PTSD 28.9 <br> • Gender: 96% male mTBI plus PTSD male .93, mTBI no PTSD 1.0 <br> • Race/Ethnicity: NR <br> • Education: NR | • Time since injury: NR, but the admission date for included subjects ranged from Aug 2004-2006, and the sample included subjects assessed for both PTSD and TBI during Sept 2005-Aug 2006. <br> • Mechanism of Injury: Mechanism for burn injury not specified. Blast injury: sustaining a combat injury caused by explosive munitions, such as an IED, RPG, Explosively Formed Projectile (EFP), mortar rounds, VBIED, and conventional grenades. <br> • Prior TBI: NR |
| Gordon, Fitzpatrick, Hilsabeck, 2011[22] | Veterans who had undergone a neuropsychological evaluation at South Texas Veterans Health Care System; selected from research database. 13/95 excluded based on an invalid TOMM score. | • Definition: LOC; PTA; normal CT and/or MRI <br> • Positive imaging: Excluded; state "uncomplicated." <br> • Citation: Kay et al., 1993 <br> • How assessed: Self-report survey, clinical interview | 82 | • Age: 49.8 (11.9) <br> • Gender: 88% male <br> • Race/Ethnicity: non-Hispanic White (52%); Hispanic (33%); African Americans (10%); Asian Americans (4%); Native Americans (1%) <br> • Education: 12.9 (2.4) yrs | • Time since injury: 20.1 (14.7) months <br> • MVA (27%); falls (20%); sports injuries (12%); industrial accidents (11%); miscellaneous accidents (11%); assaults (10%); and explosions (9%). "Most (89%) were not sustained during combat." <br> • Prior TBI: NR |
| Gottshall, Drake, Gray, et al., 2003[23] | From Feb 2000 to Nov 2000, 99 male subjects were evaluated at Camp Pendleton Concussion Clinic (presumably these 99 included 53 cases plus 46 volunteer controls). All subjects were active duty and had no premorbid history of psychiatric or substance abuse disorder. All individuals with mild TBI and a GCS of 14 were included. | • Definition: American Academy of Neurology mTBI definition, <br> • Positive imaging: NR <br> • Citation: Schubert, Herdman, & Tusa, 2001; Kay et al., 1993 <br> • How assessed: Chart review | 99, 53 | • Age: 22 (SD, NR) <br> • Gender: 100% male <br> • Race/Ethnicity: NR <br> • Education: 98% completed HS; 32% had taken some college-level courses; 4% graduated from college | • Time since injury: mean of 84 hrs post injury (range 2 hrs to 6 days, with the exception of one patient who was not seen until 10 days). <br> • Mechanism of Injury: NR <br> • Prior TBI: NR |

| Author, year | Population and sample selection | mTBI definition and associated citation reported in the study | Sample size: Total, mTBI | Demographics of mTBI group | Time since injury for mTBI group, Mean (SD); Mechanism of injury; Prior TBI |
|---|---|---|---|---|---|
| Kelly, Coldren, Parish, et al., 2012[24] | All U.S. Army soldiers in Iraq presenting for medical care within 72 hrs of a concussive event, from January to April 2009. Inclusion: 18–50, meet DoD criteria for concussion, free of cognition altering medication; have no severe psychiatric diagnosis requiring ongoing therapy (i.e., ongoing medication management by a psychiatrist), report pain not more than 7 of 10, and give consent. Excluded: prior severe TBI, moderate TBI within the previous 3 yrs, or any concussion within the previous 90 days; two cases after demonstrating poor effort on the TOMM; women due to small number of subjects (n = 3). | • Definition: DoD criteria<br>• Positive imaging: NR<br>• Citation: DoD, 2007<br>• How assessed: Self-report survey, clinical interview | 212, 66 | • Cases (n = 66) vs. controls (n = 146)<br>• Age median (IQR): 25 (22,30) vs. 25 (22,31), p = ns<br>• Gender: 100% male<br>• Race/Ethnicity, (%): p = ns white 74 vs. 70: black 6 vs. 16; Hispanic 17 vs. 8; Asian 0 vs. 1; American Indian 0 vs. 1; Pacific Islander 0 vs. 1; Other 8 vs. 6<br>• Education (%): p = 0.03; HS: 9 vs. 3; HS graduate 48 vs. 55; Some college 39 vs. 29; College graduate 3 vs. 12 | • Time since injury: NR. Cases were admitted within 72 hrs of injury; neuropsych testing administered after a full night's rest.<br>• Mechanism of Injury (%, cases only): Blast: 53%, Blow: 27%, Mixed: 9%, Unknown: 11%<br>• Prior TBI: p<0.01 0: 68 vs. 86; 1: 20 vs. 10; 2: 9 vs. 1 |
| Kennedy, Cullen, Amador, et al., 2010[25] | US military evaluated from Jan 2007-Apr 2009 at Brooke AMC, Ft Sam Houston, Lackland AFB referred to DVBIC. Excluded: moderate, severe, or penetrating TBI; those injured while deployed to OEF; more than 3 OIF deployments; female; non-blast injury mechanism; evaluation more than 12 months after injury. | • Definition: ACRM criteria; and GCS of 13-15<br>• Positive imaging: NR<br>• Citation: ACRM, 1993<br>• How assessed: Clinical interview | 274 | • Age: 28.15 (7.1) mTBI only; 25.40 (5.5) mTBI mTBI plus at least one other AIS coded injury<br>• Gender: 100% male<br>• Race/Ethnicity: NR<br>• Education: NR | • Time since injury: 12.95 (12.9), 12.63(13.4) wks<br>• Mechanism of Injury: Blast or explosion<br>• Prior TBI: NR |
| Kennedy, Leal, Lewis, et al., 2010[26] | U.S. military service members who were evaluated and diagnosed with mTBI at the San Antonio Military Medical Center from May 23, 2005 to August 31, 2009. Excluded: 97 patients who had incomplete data on the PCL-C; 89 patients with more severe TBI, and 16 with no clear date of injury. | • Definition: ACRM criteria<br>• Positive imaging: NR<br>• Citation: Kay et al., 1993<br>• How assessed: Clinical interview | 724, 586 | • Age: 27.9 (7.4)<br>• Gender: 96.7% male<br>• Race/Ethnicity: NR<br>• Education: NR | • Time since injury: Total mTBI sample: 31.3 (47.1) wks; Blast: 30.6 (45.4) wks; Non-blast: 34.1 (54.0) wks<br>• Mechanism of Injury: non-blast mTBI group: deployment-related events such as MVAs, assaults and falls and not as a direct result of a blast explosion.<br>• Prior TBI: NR |
| Lew, Pogoda Hsu, Cohen, Amick, Baker, Meterko, Vanderploeg, 2010[27] | VA patients (OEF/OIF) who screened positive for symptomatic TBI on 4-item screen, referred to polytrauma outpatient clinic, and completed 2nd level comprehensive TBI evaluation in VA polytrauma outpatient clinic (n = 200) from n = 327 who were seen at the polytrauma network site between 1/1/08 and 04/30/09. | • Definition: Positive 4-item VA TBI screen and subsequently diagnosed with TBI based on 2nd level comprehensive TBI evaluation including severity rating.<br>• Positive imaging: NR<br>• Citation: GAO, 2008 & VHA, 2007 cited for screening; Kay et al., 1993 cited for secondary clinical evaluation.<br>• How assessed: Self-report screen and follow-up clinical evaluation | 200, 131 | Note: Only age reported for mTBI sample; all other demographics reported for whole sample<br>• Age: 31.02 (9.14)<br>• Gender: 94% male<br>• Race/Ethnicity: NR<br>• Education: pre-military education = 71.7% HS or less | • Time since injury: NR<br>• Mechanism of Injury: NR<br>• Prior TBI: NR |

| Author, year | Population and sample selection | mTBI definition and associated citation reported in the study | Sample size: Total, mTBI | Demographics of mTBI group | Time since injury for mTBI group, Mean (SD); Mechanism of injury; Prior TBI |
|---|---|---|---|---|---|
| Lippa, Pasternik, Benge, & Thornton, 2010[28] | Veterans with current mTBI symptoms referred for evaluation through the VA TBI screening process. Excluded: not meeting mTBI criteria. | • Definition: LOC, or disorientation < 24 hrs<br>• Positive imaging: NR<br>• Citation: CDC, 2003<br>• How assessed: Self-report | 339 | • Age: 30.28 (7.59)<br>• Gender: 96.2% male<br>• Race/Ethnicity: 13.3% African American; 62.8% Caucasian; 20.1% Hispanic; 3.8% Other<br>• Education: 55.8% HS Diploma or equivalent; 37.5% some college; 5.6% college graduate; 1.2% other | • Time since injury: 36.72 (19.5) for last reported injury<br>• Mechanism of Injury: Blast (n = 138), non-blast (n = 56), or both (n = 145)<br>• Prior TBI: Some participants had multiple TBIs |
| Nelson, Hoelzle, Doane, et al., 2012[29] | National Guard soldiers from a Brigade Combat Team n = 41 and OEF/OIF Veterans from VA polytrauma rehabilitation and PTSD clinics n = 61. Excluded: current psychotic disorder, current/past substance abuse/dependence other than alcohol/caffeine/ nicotine, DSM-IV diagnosis prior to deployment, neurologic condition before deployment, current/ pre-deployment unstable medical condition that would likely affect brain functioning, significant risk of suicidal/homicidal behavior, and history of TBI greater than mild in severity, insufficient effort testing. | • Definition: LOC, any loss of memory for events surrounding the event, any alteration in mental state, and focal neurologic deficits, PTA<br>• Positive imaging: NR<br>• Citation: Kay et al., 1993<br>• How assessed: Participant self-reported symptoms evaluated by psychological consensus team. | 104 | * 67 participants included in Nelson et al., 2010<br>• Age: VA = 29.3 (6.3), National Guard = 35.5 (8.7)<br>• Gender: 93.3% male<br>• Race/Ethnicity: 97.1% Caucasian<br>• Education: 14.4 (2.2) yrs | • Time since injury: 177.2 (85.5) weeks since most recent blast exposure<br>• Mechanism of Injury: 84.6% blast exposed overall (regardless of mechanism of mTBI); 50% of overall sample had blast-related concussions<br>• Prior TBI: Included history of mild; 10.5 (21.7) mean number of blast exposures |
| Nelson, Hoelzle, McGuire, et al., 2010[30] | U.S. Veterans within the Midwestern region of the USA/VISN 23; Research participants were recruited consecutively at the Minneapolis VA Medical Center. Participants required to meet mTBI criteria. | • Definition: ACRM definition<br>• Positive imaging: NR<br>• Citation: Kay et al., 2003<br>• How assessed: Clinical interview | 119 | • Age: 35.5 (10.2)<br>• Gender: 93.3% male<br>• Race/Ethnicity: 93.3% Caucasian<br>• Education: 13.7 (2.3) yrs | • Time since injury: 327.0 (425.6) days (most recent concussion)<br>• Mechanism of Injury, n: Forensic or compensation context: OEF/ OIF blast, 19; non-blast, 5; OEF/ OIF non-blast, 1; non-blast n, 11; other, 8; Research context OEF/ OIF blast, 38; OEF/OIF non-blast, 37<br>• Prior TBI: NR |
| Patil, St. Andre, Crisan, et al., 2011[31] | Consecutive OEF/OIF combat Veterans with diagnosis of mTBI seen at VA PNS, June 2007-July 2009. Excluded: attending neurology appointment for reasons other than headache; mechanism of injury other than trauma. | • Definition: Based on VA/DoD Consensus-based Classification of Closed TBI Severity<br>• Positive imaging: Included. 45/56 veterans seen in neurology clinic had CT, MR or both. 40% of these with white matter changes, 30% with sinus polyps/cysts, 25% with arachnoid cysts/ vascular malformations/masses, 5% atrophy<br>• Citation: Defense and Veterans Brain Injury Center, 2006<br>• How assessed: Clinical interview, chart review | n/a, 246 | • Age: 27.9 (6.3)<br>• Gender: 92.3% male<br>• Race/Ethnicity: 85% White<br>• Education: >99% completed HS or GED | • Time since injury: NR<br>• Mean time between mTBI event and neurology visit: 3.1 yrs (data missing in 24/56 patients)<br>• Mechanism of Injury: 65% blast-exposure<br>• Prior TBI: NR |

| Author, year | Population and sample selection | mTBI definition and associated citation reported in the study | Sample size: Total, mTBI | Demographics of mTBI group | Time since injury for mTBI group, Mean (SD); Mechanism of injury; Prior TBI |
|---|---|---|---|---|---|
| Ruff, Riechers, Wang, et al., 2012[32] | OEF/OIF veterans; sought care from the VHA, Louis Stokes CVAMC. Excluded: moderate or penetrating TBI. Results reported for three groups: combat veterans with LOC, combat veterans without LOC, and then Veterans with civilian mTBI. | • Definition: An episode of TBI with LOC, AOC, and/or PTA<br>• Positive imaging: NR<br>• Citation: Malec, Brown, Liebson, et al., 2007<br>• How assessed: clinical interview | 163 *does not include 5 veterans with "probable" mTBI | Combat Veterans with LOC; combat Veterans without LOC; and then Veterans with civilian mTBI.<br>• Age: 29.2 (2.6); 30.0 (1.6); 35.1 (2.2)<br>• Gender: 92.1, 90.5, 90.5% male<br>• Race/Ethnicity: NR<br>• Education: 100% HS graduates; 8.7, 5, 9.5% college graduates | • Time since injury: NR<br>• Mechanism of Injury: Military and civilian incidents<br>• Prior TBI: NR |
| Ruff, Ruff, & Wang, 2008[33] | OEF/OIF veterans; evaluated at the VHA, Louis Stokes Department of CVAMC. Exclusions: the initial screen was not truly positive because a veteran did not understand a question; the veteran had moderate or severe TBI or had sustained penetrating TBI; TBI was not due to exposure to an explosion; and the veteran did not complete the second-level evaluation. | • Definition: LOC, any alteration in mental state following the TBI < 24 hrs, PTA<br>• Positive imaging: NR<br>• Citation: Ruff, 2005; Malec, Brown, Liebson, et al., 2007; Esselman & Uomoto, 1995; Kay et al., 1993<br>• How assessed: self-report screening tool and clinical interview | 126 | • Age: NR<br>• Gender: NR<br>• Race/Ethnicity: NR<br>• Education: NR | • Time since injury: NR<br>• Mechanism of Injury: Explosion<br>• Prior TBI: NR |
| Ruff, Ruff, & Wang, 2009[34] | OEF/OIF veterans; evaluated at the VHA, Louis Stokes Department of CVAMC. Same exclusions as Ruff, Ruff, & Wang, 2008 above. Included veterans from the previous study who had "abnormalities on neurological examination, neuropsychological testing, or both" as well as headaches." | • Definition: LOC, the duration of any alteration in mental state following the TBI < 24 hrs, PTA<br>• Positive imaging: NR<br>• Citation: Kushner, 1998; Ruff, 2005; Malec, Brown, Liebson, et al., 2007; Esselman & Uomoto, 1995; Kay et al., 1993<br>• How assessed: self-report screening tool and clinical interview | 74 | Note: Subpopulation from the Ruff et al., 2008 study also reported<br>• Age: 29.4 (2.9)<br>• Gender: 95% male<br>• Race/Ethnicity: NR<br>• Education: NR | • Time since injury: NR<br>• Mechanism of Injury: Explosion<br>• Prior TBI: NR |
| Schiehser, Delis, Filoteo, et al., 2011[35] | Active duty noncombat, nondeployed service members with mild TBI. Recruited thru local DVBIC; actual recruitment procedures not specified | • Definition: LOC; GCS score between 13 and 15; and/or PTA<br>• Positive imaging: Excluded (classified as moderate TBI)<br>• Citation: NR<br>• How assessed: "Self-report" | 66, 44 | Note: mild and moderate TBI populations combined<br>• Age: NR<br>• Gender: NR<br>• Race/Ethnicity: NR<br>• Education: NR | • Time since injury: 38.3 (11.8) days<br>• Mechanism of Injury: Blunt force<br>• Prior TBI: Excluded |
| Spencer, Drag, Walker, et al., 2010[36] | Referrals to the TBI Clinic at the VA Ann Arbor Health Care System for a more comprehensive medical evaluation which included a neuropsych assessment. Excluded: inconsistent effort on neuropsych testing as evidenced by a score of 8 or below on the Rey 15-item Memory Test; seen as part of a C and P; exceeded criteria for mild TBI | • Definition: screened positive for possible head injury on standard VA clinical reminder consisting of PCS<br>• Positive imaging: NR<br>• Citation: NR<br>• How assessed: Clinical Interview | 105 | • Age: 29.8 (8.2)<br>• Gender: NR<br>• Race/Ethnicity: NR<br>• Education: 12.9 (1.4) yrs | • Time since injury: NR<br>• Mechanism of Injury: NR<br>• Prior TBI: NR |

| Author, year | Population and sample selection | mTBI definition and associated citation reported in the study | Sample size: Total, mTBI | Demographics of mTBI group | Time since injury for mTBI group, Mean (SD); Mechanism of injury; Prior TBI |
|---|---|---|---|---|---|
| Swick, Honzel, Larsen, et al., 2012[37] | Combat Veterans diagnosed with PTSD. Controls were recruited primarily through advertisements. Excluded: significant medical disease, severe psychiatric problems (such as schizophrenia or bipolar disorder), active substance abuse, visual deficits, or history of other neurological events. | • Definition: VA/DoD Clinical Practice Guidelines<br>• Positive imaging: NR<br>• Citation: The Management of Concussion/mTBI Working Group, 2009<br>• How assessed: Clinical interview | 73, 30 | • Age: 32.3 (7.5)<br>• Gender: 97% male<br>• Race/Ethnicity: NR<br>• Education: 13.6 (1.2) yrs | • Time since injury: 3.8 (1.5) yrs postdeployment; time since injury NR<br>• Mechanism of Injury: NR<br>• Prior TBI: Yes, some |
| Theeler & Erickson, 2009[38] | US Army soldiers who were evaluated between Jan and June 2006 in the Neurology Clinic at Madigan Army Medical Center for chronic headaches following a 12-month combat tour in Iraq. Soldiers were eligible if they experienced headaches during deployment and continued to experience headaches for 3 or more months after returning from Iraq. | • Definition: DVBIC Working Group on the Acute Management of Mild Traumatic Brain Injury in Military Operational Settings criteria<br>• Positive imaging: NR<br>• Citation: DVBIC Working Group on the Acute Management of Mild Traumatic Brain Injury in Military Operational Settings Clinical Practice Guideline and Recommendations, ND<br>• How assessed: Chart review | 81, 33 | • Age: 29.1<br>• Gender: 80% male<br>• Race/Ethnicity: NR<br>• Education: NR | • Time since injury: NR<br>• Mechanism of Injury: Of the n = 33 (41%) with head or neck trauma: 15% blunt trauma, 18% other explosive, 67% blast<br>• Prior TBI: Multiple head or neck injuries occurred in 6 soldiers |
| Toblin, Riviere, Thomas, et al., 2012[39] | Soldiers from 3 U.S. infantry brigade combat teams surveyed 6 months post-deployment during Nov-Dec 2008, deployed to Iraq or Afghanistan for at least one month. 50% of all soldiers from participating units were present during recruitment phase. Excluded: 10 soldiers who reported moderate or severe TBI | • Definition: Combat injury was grouped into no injury, non-mTBI injury, mTBI with AOC but no LOC, and mTBI with LOC.<br>• Positive imaging: NR<br>• Citation: Hoge et al., 2008<br>• How assessed: Self-report survey | 1522, NR | • Age: NR<br>• Gender: NR<br>• Race/Ethnicity: NR<br>• Education: NR | • Time since injury: NR<br>• Mechanism of Injury: NR<br>• Prior TBI: NR |

22

## SUMMARY OF FINDINGS

In general, we found that, though cognitive, physical, and mental health symptoms were frequently reported by Veterans/military members following mTBI, there was little evidence that symptoms were more common in those with mTBI than those without mTBI. However, the evidence base is weakened by inconsistent findings, methodologic shortcomings of many studies, and variation in outcomes considered and outcome measurement approaches. We grouped findings into categories according to our key questions; though some outcomes could have been included in multiple categories (e.g., sleep), we chose to categorize outcomes as commonly reported in the literature, and report specific outcomes within each category individually for clarity. Findings by outcome categories are reported in detail in the following sections.

## COGNITIVE FUNCTIONING RESULTS

### Summary of Cognitive Functioning Results

We found 17 studies reporting cognitive outcomes for those with mTBI. Overall, few studies found an association between mTBI and cognitive deficits. The strength of evidence is very low because of poor and incomplete reporting of data and sampling procedures, lack of time-since-injury information, and because most studies were unblinded and single-center.

The studies reporting cognitive outcomes reported mean scores rather than proportions of individuals with impaired scores, making estimates of prevalence of cognitive impairment impossible. The best approximation of prevalence of impairment comes from studies reporting standardized scores which can be associated with impairment below certain cutoffs, and cognitive results should ideally be adjusted for pre-morbid functioning since the most accurate assessment of impairment reflects intra-individual change over time. We report estimates of impairment based on mean standardized scores, when available, and none of the included studies provided information on pre-morbid functioning such that change from baseline could be assessed at the intra-individual level. Though the majority of studies reported mean standardized scores within normal limits, the nature of mean score reporting is such that individuals comprising those means may have scored significantly above or below the mean. Therefore, though overall scores may be within normal limits, it is likely that some individuals obtained scores indicative of impairment, and individual variation should be kept in mind when interpreting findings.

There were studies that found mTBI patients had deficits in visuospatial abilities, attention/concentration, and total/cross-domain composite scores as compared to patients without mTBI. However, even within each of these subdomains, findings were inconsistent across studies. In nearly all studies, scores for each of the subscales fell within normal limits, suggesting no clinically significant impairment in the group as a whole. Because studies did not report the proportion of patients scoring below normal range for each of the subscales, it is unclear whether there may have been subgroups of mTBI patients with cognitive deficits. Of note, single studies reported that mTBI patients within 10 days of injury and those undergoing disability evaluation had low processing speed scores.

It is difficult to draw overall conclusions about which factors, in addition to mTBI, are independently associated with cognitive test performance since studies evaluated a variety of different factors and there were inconsistent findings among them. Individual studies suggested that impaired cognitive test performance was associated with comorbid mental health diagnosis, time since injury of less than 10 days, self-reported cognitive complaints, and experiencing loss or alteration of consciousness at the time of injury. One study found that Veterans who participated in a headache intervention demonstrated better overall cognitive functioning post-intervention than those who did not participate in the intervention.

Prevalence estimates of self-reported cognitive complaints were not reported in the included studies. Potential risk factors for more severe self-reported cognitive problems include having an additional injury, LOC or PTA at the time of injury, being service connected, and having an Axis I mental health disorder.

The following table summarizes the evidence on cognitive outcomes, which is then followed by detailed results descriptions for each cognitive domain.

**Table 2. Summary of Evidence for Cognitive Functioning Outcomes Associated with mTBI in Veteran and Military Populations**

| Domain (number of studies) | Key Question 1: Estimates of Prevalence and Impairment (number of studies) | Key Question 1: Statistically Significant Deficits Compared to Controls (number of studies) | Key Question 2: Statistically Significant Potential Risk or Protective Factors (number of studies) |
|---|---|---|---|
| Language Abilities and General Fund of Verbal Knowledge (8) | Mean scores were within normal limits (7) | No (3) | No: Axis I disorder (2)<br>No: Blast exposure (1)<br>No: Disability/C&P Evaluation (1)<br>No: LOC or PTA (1) |
| Visuospatial Abilities (6) | Mean scores were within normal limits (2) | Yes (1)<br>No (1) | Yes Risk: Axis I disorder (1)<br>No: Axis I disorder (3)<br>No: Blast exposure (1)<br>No: Self-reported cognitive problems (1) |
| Memory (11) | Mean scores were within normal limits (5) | No (3)<br>Yes (2 studies on same population; differences only significant within 5 days of injury) | Yes Risk: Time since injury 72 hours (1)<br>Yes Risk: Axis I disorder (1)<br>Mixed Risk: Axis I disorder (2)<br>Mixed Risk: Self-reported cognitive problems (1)<br>Mixed Risk: Time since injury 5 days (1)<br>No: Axis I disorder (1)<br>No: Blast exposure (2)<br>No: Disability/C&P Evaluation (1)<br>No: LOC or PTA (1)<br>No: Service connection (1)<br>No: Time since injury 10 days (1) |
| Attention/Concentration (8) | Mean scores were within normal limits (2) | No (2)<br>Yes (3) | Yes Risk: Time since injury 72 hours (1)<br>Mixed Risk: Axis I disorder (1)<br>No: Axis I disorder (1)<br>No: Blast exposure (1)<br>No: Disability/C&P Evaluation (1)<br>No: LOC or AOC (1)<br>No: Service connection (1)<br>No: Self-reported cognitive problems (1)<br>No: Time since injury 5-10 days (1) |

| Domain (number of studies) | Key Question 1: Estimates of Prevalence and Impairment (number of studies) | Key Question 1: Statistically Significant Deficits Compared to Controls (number of studies) | Key Question 2: Statistically Significant Potential Risk or Protective Factors (number of studies) |
|---|---|---|---|
| Processing Speed (9) | Mean scores were within normal limits; exceptions were scores below expected limits for some participants evaluated for disability/C&P and < 10 days since injury. (4) | No (5) | Yes Risk: Disability/C&P Evaluation (1)<br>Yes Risk: Time since injury 5 days (1)<br>No: Axis I disorders (3)<br>No: Blast exposure (1)<br>No: LOC or PTA (1)<br>No: Time since injury 10 days (1) |
| Executive Functioning (7) | Mean scores were within normal limits (4) | No (2) | No: Axis I disorder (3)<br>No: Blast exposure (1)<br>No: Disability/C&P Evaluation (1)<br>No: LOC or PTA (1) |
| Effort/Motivation (1) | Mean scores were within normal limits (1) | No (1) | Yes Risk: Disability/C&P Evaluation (1) |
| Total and Cross-Domain Composite Scores (9) | Mean scores were within normal limits (2) | No (2)<br>Yes (1) | Yes Protective: Participation in headache intervention (1)<br>Yes Risk: Disability/C&P Evaluation (1)<br>Yes Risk: LOC or AOC (1)<br>No: Blast exposure (1) |
| Self-reported Cognitive Deficits (7) | NR | NR | Yes Protective: Additional injury (1)<br>Yes Risk: LOC or PTA (1)<br>Yes Risk: Service Connection (1)<br>Yes Risk: Axis I disorder (4)<br>No: Axis I disorder (1)<br>No: Blast exposure (1) |

*Note.* The impairment summary is based on average scores for groups with mTBI, and does not reflect individual variation in scores which could include some impairment for a certain proportion of participants. "Mixed" results indicate both significant and non-significant results for multiple assessments of the same outcome in a single study.

## Language Abilities and General Fund of Verbal Knowledge

Key Question 1: We found eight primary studies that assessed this domain of cognitive functioning using the Repeatable Battery for the Assessment of Neuropsychological Status (RBANS): Language subtest, the Shipley Institute of Living Scale Vocabulary subtest, the Wechsler Adult Intelligence Scale-Third Edition (WAIS-III) Information subtest, and the Wechsler Adult Test of Adult Reading (WTAR).[10,11,16,18,20,22,29,30] The results abstracted from these studies are found in Appendix E, Table 1a. Three studies examined outcomes compared to a non-TBI group from the same population, describing similar performance across groups.[18,29,30] All of the three studies reported standardized scores, and all of the mean scores fell within normal limits for language abilities and general fund of verbal knowledge, suggesting that, on average, clinically significant impairment in this domain is not associated with mTBI. None of the studies reported proportions of patients who obtained impaired scores on tests of language abilities and general fund of verbal knowledge.

Key Question 2: One study examined differences between Veterans with a history of mTBI who were obtaining testing as part of a C and P evaluation (i.e., a disability evaluation associated with potential financial gain) versus those recruited in a research context, and reported no significant differences between the groups.[30] A study by the same group of authors examined the effect of having an Axis I disorder on two different tests assessing language abilities and general fund of verbal knowledge, and both tests indicated non-significant differences between groups.[29] Similarly, studies examining the possible effect of PTSD diagnosis or mental health diagnosis other than PTSD[22] and LOC and/or PTA at the time of injury (compared to solely experiencing alteration of consciousness)[20] both reported non-significant group differences. One study reported non-significant differences between Veterans with mTBI who were exposed to blast versus those who were not exposed to blast.[16]

## Visuospatial Abilities

Key Question 1: Six primary studies reported visuospatial outcomes using the RBANS: Visuospatial/Constructional subscale; Rey Complex Figure Test (RCFT); a study-specific Visual Organization/Processing factor; and the WAIS-III: Block Design subtest (Appendix E, Table 1b).[16,18,20,22,29,36] In the studies that directly compared mTBI with non-TBI participants from the same population, groups performed similarly on two measures of visuospatial abilities (WAIS-III Block Design and RCFT Figure Copy), though the mTBI group performed significantly worse than participants without mTBI on the RBANS Visuospatial/Constructional subscale.[18,29] All of the mean standardized scores reported in these studies are within normal limits for visuospatial abilities.

Key Question 2: Studies examining the effects of Axis I disorders,[29] PTSD diagnosis,[22] or mental health diagnosis other than PTSD[22] reported equivalent results across groups. Contrary to these results, another research group examined the association between mental health variables including PTSD, depression, and anxiety with a visual organization/processing factor score, and reported significant negative correlations between visuospatial abilities and both self-reported PTSD and depression symptoms, but non-significant differences for service connection and LOC or PTA at the time of injury.[20] One study reported non-significant differences based on blast exposure.[16] Finally, a study examining self-reported cognitive deficits found no significant association with objective visuospatial test results.[36]

## Memory

Key Question 1: We found 11 primary studies that assessed this domain of cognitive functioning using the Automated Neuropsychological Assessment Metrics (ANAM): Code Substitution Delayed (CDD) and Matching to Sample (MSP) subtests; Brief Visuospatial Memory Test Revised (BVMT-R): Total Recall and Delayed Recall subtests; the California Verbal Learning Test Second Edition (CVLT-II): Trials 1-5, Short Delay Free Recall, and Long Delay Free Recall subscales; a study-specific Memory Composite Score; a study-specific Memory Factor; the RBANS Story Memory Immediate Recall, Story Memory Delayed Recall, Immediate Memory, and Delayed Memory subtests; the RCFT: Immediate Recall and Delayed Recall subtests; and the WAIS-III: Digit Symbol Coding subtest (Appendix E, Table 1c).[11,15,16,18,20,22,24,29,30,35,36] Five studies examined outcomes compared to a non-TBI group from the same population, reporting similar results across groups in most cases.[15,18,24,29,30] The notable exception was from two studies by the same group of authors and the same patient population which reported significant group differences on both 72 hour assessments, one of the two 5 day assessments, and neither of the 10 day assessments.[15,24] In these two studies, the participants were assessed by the ANAM subtests, and the assessments were conducted within 72 hours, 5 days, and 10 days of injury; the rest of the comparisons were between populations with longer time since injury, and using assessment tools other than the ANAM. Of the studies which reported standardized scores on assessments, all of the mean scores fell within normal limits for memory functioning; none of the studies reported proportions of patients who obtained impaired scores on tests of memory.[11,18,20,29,30]

Key Question 2: As noted above, two studies reported ANAM outcomes at specific times following mTBI event; these studies report significant deficits in memory on the majority of ANAM subtests at 72 hours and 5 days following injury.[15,24] These same studies also report comparisons with controls after 10 days following injury, and notably these latter results are both non-significant. One study reported non-significant differences between Veterans with mTBI who were exposed to blast versus those who were not exposed to blast in terms of their immediate and delayed memory test performance.[16] One study examined differences between Veterans with mTBI who were obtaining testing as part of a C and P evaluation versus those recruited in a research context, reporting non-significant differences between groups.[30] A study by the same group of authors examined the effect of having an Axis I disorder on three tests assessing memory, and two out of three assessment results indicated non-significant differences between individuals with mTBI who did and did not have an Axis I disorder.[29] One study examined the effect of mental health diagnosis other than PTSD on memory outcomes, and found similar results across groups.[22] Two studies examined the effect of PTSD on memory outcomes. One of these studies did not report p-values, though results for four out of five memory tests were worse for those with a diagnosis of PTSD.[22] The other study reported a significant negative relationship between scores on a self-report PTSD symptom inventory and a composite memory score.[20] This latter study also reported a non-significant association for self-reported depression and service connection with memory test results, though self-reported anxiety was significantly related to memory functioning.[20] A study examining self-reported cognitive deficits found no significant correlation between memory test results and self-reported cognitive deficits for two out of three tests.[36] One study examined the impact of blast exposure and reported no significant differences between groups.[11] Finally, one study reported similar results across groups based on mTBI with LOC and/or PTA at the time of injury compared to those with mTBI who only reported alteration of consciousness at the time of the mTBI event.[20]

## Attention/Concentration

Key Question 1: We found eight primary studies that assessed this domain of cognitive functioning using the ANAM: Mathematical Processing (MTH) subtest; the RBANS: Attention subscale; study-specific Visual and Verbal Attention factor scores; and the WAIS-III and WAIS-IV: Digit Span subtest scores (Appendix E, Table 1d).[15,16,18,20,24,29,30,36] In five studies that compared mTBI directly with non-mTBI controls, findings varied with the metric used. The mTBI group performed similarly to a non-TBI comparison group on the WAIS-IV Digit Span measures of attention in two studies,[29,30] In other studies, participants with mTBI performed worse on the RBANS subtest and on the ANAM subtest, but deficits noted at 72 hours diminished with time.[15,18,24] As with other outcomes, mean scores fell within normal limits for attention/concentration abilities.[29,30]

Key Question 2: Seven studies reported results separately for mTBI groups with and without potential risk or protective factors.[15,16,20,24,29,30,36] As noted with other cognitive outcomes, significant deficits in attention/concentration at 72 hours following injury diminished to non-significant differences 5 and 10 days following injury.[15,24] One study reported non-significant differences in attention based on blast exposure.[16] The study that compared mTBI participants in a research setting with a forensic setting (i.e., a setting in which patients were evaluated for potential compensation) found non-significant differences in attention/concentration, in contrast with other outcomes for which participants in the forensic setting performed worse.[30] Having an Axis I disorder in addition to mTBI did not emerge as a significant factor on attention/ concentration outcomes.[29] A study that examined the possible effects of PTSD, anxiety, and depression on attention and concentration outcomes reported significant associations between worse visual, but not verbal attention for depression and anxiety, and significant negative associations between both visual and verbal attention for PTSD.[20] Service connection was non-significantly associated with verbal and visual attention.[20] Participants with LOC and/or PTA following TBI had similar results on attention/concentration compared with those who did not have these immediate sequelae.[20] WAIS-IV Digit Span test results were not significantly correlated with self-reported cognitive deficits in one study.[36]

## Processing Speed

Key Question 1: We found nine primary studies that assessed processing using the ANAM: Code Substitution (CDS), Procedural Reaction Time (PRT) subtest, and Simple Reaction Time (SRT) subtest; reaction time on a Go/NoGo task; Stroop Color & Word Test: Color and Word subtests; the Trail Making Test Part A; and the WAIS-III: Digit Symbol Coding subtest (Appendix E, Table 1e).[11,15,20,22,24,29,30,36,37] Five studies examined outcomes compared to a non-TBI group from the same population.[15,24,29,30,37] In three of these studies, the mTBI group performed similarly to a non-TBI comparison group on multiple measures of processing speed.[29,30,37] By contrast, two studies conducted in the same patient population using the ANAM observed processing speed deficits soon after injury (72 hours and 5 days), although statistically significant differences between cases and controls were not detected upon longer term follow-up (10 days after injury).[15,24]

Key Question 2: As noted above, two studies report significant deficits in processing speed on the majority of ANAM subtests at 72 hours and 5 days following injury, but non-significant differences 10 days after injury.[15,24] One study examined differences between Veterans with mTBI who were obtaining testing as part of a C and P evaluation compared with Veterans with mTBI who were recruited in a research context, describing worse processing speed performance on all four tests examined by those obtaining a C & P evaluation.[30] Studies examining Axis I disorders,[29] PTSD diagnosis,[22] mental health problems other than PTSD,[22] self-reported cognitive deficits,[36] blast exposure,[11] and LOC and/or PTA[20] all reported equivalent results across compared groups.

## Executive Functioning

Key Question 1: We found seven primary studies that assessed this domain of cognitive functioning using the Controlled Oral Word Association (COWA) test, the Stroop Color and Word Test Color-Word subscale, the Trail Making Test Part B, and an Executive Functioning Composite test score (Appendix E, Table 1f).[11,20,22,29,35,36] Two studies by the same group of authors examined outcomes compared to a non-TBI group from the same population.[29,30] In these studies, the mTBI group performed similarly to a non-TBI comparison group on multiple measures of executive functioning. Of the four studies reporting standardized scores, all of the mean scores fell within normal limits for executive functioning; none of the studies reported proportions of patients who obtained impaired scores on tests of executive functioning.

Key Question 2: One study examined differences between mTBI Veterans who were obtaining testing as part of a C and P evaluation (i.e., a disability evaluation associated with potential financial gain) versus those recruited in a research context, reporting no significant differences between groups.[30] One study examined the effect of having an Axis I disorder, and all results were non-significant.[29] Similarly, another study examined the possible effect of PTSD diagnosis or mental health diagnosis other than PTSD on executive functioning outcomes, and found non-significant differences between groups.[22] A study examining self-reported cognitive deficits found no significant association with executive functioning test results.[36] One study on blast exposure reported no significant group differences.[11] Finally, one study reported non-significant group differences based on mTBI with LOC and/or PTA at time of injury compared to those with mTBI who did not have these immediate sequelae.[20]

## Effort/Motivation

Key Question 1: We found one primary study that assessed effort and motivation on cognitive tests using the CVLT-II: Forced Choice subtest, an Effort Failures composite; the Rey 15 Item test (Rey FIT): Combination test, the Victoria Symptom Validity Test (VSVT); and the WAIS-III: Reliable Digit Span subtest (Appendix E, Table 1g).[30] This study did not report comparisons between those with and without mTBI (Appendix E, Table 1g).[30]

Key Question 2: The same study also examined differences between Veterans with mTBI who were obtaining testing as part of a C and P evaluation (i.e., a disability evaluation associated with potential financial gain; n = 24) versus those with mTBI who were recruited in a research context (n = 38).[30] Veterans tested in the context of a disability evaluation scored worse on every measure of effort and motivation administered, and five out of the seven outcomes reported were statistically significant.[30]

## Total and Cross-Domain Composite Scores

Key Question 1: We found nine primary studies that assessed cognitive functioning across domains using an Attention/Processing Speed composite score; "positive neurological and/ or neuropsychological findings," Montreal Cognitive Assessment (MOCA); Overall Test Battery Mean; RBANS: Total Score; WAIS-III: Vocabulary, Information, Matrix Reasoning, Block Design Subscales; and WAIS-IV: all subtests (Appendix E, Table 1h).[16,18,22,29,30,32-35] Three studies examined outcomes compared to a non-TBI group.[18,29,30] In two of these studies,[29,30] there were no significant differences between mTBI and non-mTBI participants on Overall Test Battery Mean scores, though one study[18] reported significantly lower RBANS total scores for mTBI participants. Of the two studies reporting standardized scores on assessments, all of the mean scores fell within normal limits for cognitive functioning; none of the studies reported proportions of patients who obtained total or composite scores indicative of impaired cognitive functioning.[29,30]

Key Question 2: One study reported non-significant differences in RBANS total score between Veterans with mTBI who were exposed to blast versus those who were not exposed to blast.[16] One study examined differences between Veterans with mTBI who were obtaining testing as part of a C and P evaluation (i.e., a disability evaluation associated with potential financial gain) versus those with mTBI who were recruited in a research context, reporting significantly lower Overall Test Battery Mean scores for evaluations linked to potential financial gain.[30] A study by the same group of authors examined the effect of having an Axis I disorder, and results indicated non-significant differences between the groups.[29] Similarly, another group of authors investigated the effect of having PTSD or a mental health diagnosis other than PTSD, and reported similar cognitive functioning across groups.[22] Another study examined the possible effects of a headache intervention involving sleep hygiene, Prazosin, headache and pain education, and group therapy.[34] This study indicated that completion of the intervention was associated with significantly higher MOCA scores. The same group of authors also reported that MOCA scores were significantly lower for Veterans who experienced LOC compared to those who did not experience LOC.[32] Finally, another study by this same groups of authors reported a significant association between obtaining positive neurological or neuropsychological test results and the number of blast exposures resulting in LOC, as well as an association with the number of blast exposures resulting in either LOC or AOC.[33]

### Self-Reported Cognitive Problems

Key Question 1: Seven primary studies examined self-reported cognitive problems including self-reported blackouts; confusion; Frontal Systems Behavioral Scale (FrSBe): Subjective Executive Dysfunction pre- to post-injury change; memory problems; and Neurobehavioral Symptom Inventory (NSI): concentration, decision-making, memory, and slowed thinking/ organization items and cognitive cluster score (Appendix E, Table 1i).[12,13,17,20,25,29,35] We found no studies reporting prevalence estimates or comparisons with a non-mTBI control group.

Key Question 2: One study examining the effects of Axis I disorders reported non-significant differences between groups,[29] and another described non-significant differences for those with and without blast exposure.[12] Four studies examined self-reported cognitive problems on the NSI and their relationship to anxiety,[20] depression,[20] PTSD,[12,17,20] service connection,[20] and presence of LOC and/or PTA at the time of injury,[20] and all describe significantly worse symptoms reported by participants with mTBI with these potential risk factors. Finally, one study described having an additional injury being significantly correlated with fewer self-reported cognitive complaints.[25]

## PHYSICAL HEALTH RESULTS

### Summary of Physical Health Results

We found 17 studies reporting physical health outcomes for those with mTBI. Low strength evidence suggests that self-reported physical symptoms are associated with mTBI. This body of evidence is comprised entirely of low quality studies generally limited by poor and incomplete reporting of data and sampling procedures, lack of time-since-injury information, and lack of blinding of those conducting outcomes assessments; most studies were also single-center.

Studies included in this report suggest that symptoms reported by those with mTBI include headaches, pain, vestibular symptoms, hearing and vision problems, nausea or loss of appetite, and neurologic symptoms. One study reported that the prevalence of neurology referrals for headaches was 33.3% for Veterans with mTBI, though no other physical health studies reported prevalence estimates for these outcomes. It is also unclear whether mTBI directly contributes to the prevalence or severity of physical health symptoms, as only two studies included a comparison group of participants without mTBI. Self-reported symptom severity ranges widely across individuals and many of the reported physical health outcomes are based solely on responses to an individual item from the NSI, a general post-concussive symptom inventory. Additionally, inconsistent information on risk and protective factors provides insufficient evidence to make strong conclusions about potentially moderating factors for self-reported physical health outcomes.

The following table summarizes the evidence on physical health outcomes, which is then followed by detailed results descriptions for each physical health domain.

**Table 3. Summary of Evidence for Physical Health Outcomes Associated with mTBI in Veteran and Military Populations**

| Domain (number of studies) | Key Question 1: Estimates of Prevalence and Impairment (number of studies) | Key Question 1: Statistically Significant Deficits Compared to Controls (number of studies) | Key Question 2: Statistically Significant Potential Risk or Protective Factors (number of studies) |
|---|---|---|---|
| Headaches (10) | Prevalence of neurology referrals for headache = 33.3%. (1)<br><br>Average self-reported headache severity = "moderate-severe" (1)<br><br>Average headache pain = 4.33 on a scale of 0-10 (1) | NR | Yes Protective: Additional injury (1)<br>Yes Protective: Headache intervention (1)<br>Mixed Risk: Axis I disorder (2)<br>No: Blast exposure (2)<br>Yes Risk: Positive neurological or neuropsychological findings (1)<br>Yes Risk: Referral to neurology clinic for headaches (1) |
| Pain (2) | Median pain = 3.5 on a scale of 0-10 (1) | Yes: Average pain severity (1) | NR |
| Vestibular (6) | Average vestibular symptom severity = mild-moderate (1) | Mixed (1) | Yes Risk: 1-3 weeks following injury (1)<br>Mixed Risk: 4 weeks following injury (1)<br>Mixed Risk: Axis I disorders (2)<br>Yes Protective: Additional injury (1)<br>No: Blast exposure (1) |
| Vision (5) | Average vision-related symptom severity = mild-moderate (1) | NR | Mixed Risk: Axis I disorders (3)<br>Yes Protective: Additional injury (1)<br>No: Blast exposure (1) |
| Hearing (5) | Average hearing-related symptom severity = moderate (1) | NR | Mixed Risk: Axis I disorders (3)<br>Mixed Protective: Additional injury (1)<br>Mixed Risk: Blast exposure (1) |
| Nausea/Appetite (5) | Average appetite/ nausea-related symptom severity = mild-moderate (1) | NR | Mixed Risk: Axis I disorders (3)<br>Mixed Protective: Additional injury (1)<br>No: Blast exposure (1) |
| Neurological (5) | Average numbness or tingling severity = mild-moderate (1) | NR | Yes Risk: PTSD (2)<br>No: Additional injury (1)<br>No: Blast exposure (1)<br>Yes Risk: LOC (1) |

*Note.* The impairment summary is based on average scores for groups with mTBI, and does not reflect individual variation in scores which could include some impairment for a certain proportion of participants. "Mixed" results indicate both significant and non-significant results for multiple assessments of the same outcome in a single study.

## Headaches

Key Question 1: We found 10 primary studies that reported headache outcomes for Veterans and members of the military including self-reported headaches, headache days per month, headache duration, headache frequency, headache pain level or severity, headache type, time since injury of initiation of headaches, worsening of pre-trauma headaches, headache referral, headache medication overuse, Migraine Disability Assessment Score (MIDAS), Headache Impact Test (HIT-6) score, and NSI: Headache item (Appendix E, Table 2a).[12,13,16,17,25,29,31,33,34,38] One study without a comparison group reported prevalence of neurology referrals for headache in an mTBI population was 33.3%.[31] Another study reported an average NSI headache item scores between 1.45-2.71, corresponding to a self-report of headache severity in the moderate range.[25] Finally, one study reported average headache pain of 4.33 on a scale of 0-10 for Veterans with mTBI.[33] All other prevalence estimates and comparisons with a non-mTBI population reported in the included studies were based on populations selected because they experienced headaches, and therefore prevalence estimates are not accurate for a general mTBI population.

Key Question 2: A study comparing a similar population of Veterans with history of mTBI who also had at least one additional injury reported that additional injury is, in fact, a protective factor for experiencing headaches, reporting that those with additional injuries reported significantly lower NSI headache item severity than those without.[25] Another study investigating the effects of a headache intervention found that following completion of this intervention, Veterans reported decreased headache frequency and severity compared to a comparison group who did not complete the intervention.[34] One study reported non-significant differences in headache impact based on blast exposure.[16] One study reported a non-significant relationship between Axis I disorder and headaches.[29] All other studies investigating possible risk and protective factors reported statistically significant risk associated with blast exposure,[12] PTSD,[12,17] positive neurological or neuropsychological findings,[33] and referral to neurology clinic for headaches.[31]

## Pain

Key Question 1: We found only two studies documenting outcomes related to pain using self-reported pain in the past 30 days, and self-reported pain on a 0-10 scale (Appendix E, Table 2b).[9,27] Only one study compared pain to a non-mTBI population, describing statistically significant differences in median pain scores of 3.5/10 for the participants with mTBI and 2.0/10 for those without mTBI.[9]

Key Question 2: Neither included study provided data related to this key question.

## Vestibular

Key Question 1: We found six primary studies reporting vestibular outcomes including disorientation, dizziness, Dizziness Handicap Inventory (DHI) scores, Dynamic Visual Acuity Test (DVAT) scores, imbalance, and NSI: Feeling Dizzy, Loss of Balance, and Poor Coordination item scores (Appendix E, Table 2c).[12,13,17,23,25,29] Ranges of mean scores on vestibular NSI items ranged from 1.32-1.47 for mTBI populations, corresponding to mild-moderate symptom severity.[13] One study compared DHI and DVAT scores to non-mTBI populations, reporting significantly more vestibular symptoms in mTBI groups at 1, 2, 3, and 4 weeks following injury for DHI and 1 week but not 4 weeks following injury for DVAT.[23]

Key Question 2: As noted above, one study reported that significantly worse DVAT scores for the mTBI group became non-significantly different from those of non-mTBI controls after 4 weeks following injury.[23] Two studies reported non-significant differences in vestibular outcomes for those with Axis I disorders[29] or blast exposure.[12] Three studies reported that PTSD[12,17] and additional injury were significantly associated with worse self-reported vestibular symptoms in Veterans with mTBI.

## Vision

Key Question 1: We found five primary studies reporting vision-related outcomes including "photophobia" and NSI: Vision Problems and Sensitivity to Light item scores (Appendix E, Table 2d).[12,13,17,25,29] Ranges of mean scores on vision-related NSI items ranged from 1.51-1.72 for mTBI populations, corresponding to mild-moderate symptom severity.[13] No studies compared mTBI to non-mTBI populations.

Key Question 2: Two studies reported non-significant differences for those exposed to blast,[12] and those with Axis I disorders.[29] Four studies reported significantly worse self-reported vision-related outcomes for those with PTSD[12,17] and additional injury.[25]

## Hearing

Key Question 1: We found five primary studies reporting hearing-related outcomes including tinnitus, "phonophobia," and NSI: Hearing Difficulty and Sensitivity to Noise item scores (Appendix E, Table 2e).[12,13,17,25,29] Average self-reported hearing difficulty and sensitivity to noise were in the moderate range.[13] No studies compared mTBI to non-mTBI populations.

Key Question 2: Two studies investigating the association of blast exposure[12] and additional injury[25] with hearing-related outcomes reported significant findings for sensitivity to noise, but not for hearing difficulty. One study reported non-significant differences for those with Axis I disorders.[29] Two studies reported significantly worse self-reported hearing-related outcomes for those with PTSD.[12,17]

## Neurological

Key Question 1: We found five primary studies reporting neurological outcomes including neurological deficits based on examination, and NSI: Numbness or Tingling item score (Appendix E, Table 2f).[12,13,17,25,32] Average self-reported numbness or tingling was of mild-moderate severity.[13] No studies compared populations with mTBI to those without mTBI.

Key Question 2: One study investigating the association of blast exposure with the NSI item score described non-significant group differences,[12] as did a study on presence of additional injury.[25] Two studies reported significantly worse NSI numbness or tingling score for those with PTSD.[12,17] Finally, one study reported that Veterans with LOC at the time of injury were significantly more likely to obtain positive neurological exam findings than those without LOC.[32]

## Nausea/Appetite

Key Question 1: We found five primary studies reporting outcomes related to appetite and nausea including self-reported nausea, and NSI: Loss of Appetite, Change in Taste or Smell, and Nausea item scores (Appendix E, Table 2g).[12,13,17,25,29] Average self-reported change in taste or smell, nausea, and loss of appetite ranged from mild to moderate in severity.[13] No studies compared populations with mTBI to those without mTBI.

Key Question 2: One study reported that having an additional injury was a protective factor on two NSI items, but non-significantly related to the NSI item assessing change in taste or smell.[25] Two studies investigating the association of blast exposure[12] and presence of an Axis I disorder reported non-significant group differences for items assessing nausea, appetite, and changes in taste and smell.[29] Two studies reported significantly worse self-reported appetite and nausea-related outcomes for those with PTSD.[12,17]

# MENTAL HEALTH RESULTS

## Summary of Mental Health Results

Twenty studies reported mental health outcomes for Veterans or members of the military with mTBI. Mental health outcomes varied greatly in terms of methods of assessment, ranging from lengthy clinical interviews based on diagnostic criteria, to single-item, self-report screeners. Overall, this body of literature provides low strength evidence, as it is based on studies with many methodological limitations.

Studies included in this review suggest that there are high rates of comorbid mental health disorders and symptoms for those with mTBI. Notably, studies examined different, sometimes overlapping mental health outcomes (e.g., some studies examined only PTSD, while others reported combined mental health outcomes such as "any Axis I disorder." Rates of Axis I disorders ranged from 50-78% in two studies; single studies reported that reported that the rate of PTSD was 45%, alcohol abuse/dependence was 28%, drug abuse/dependence was 9% suicidal ideation was 25%, suicidal intent was 7%, and past suicide attempts was 4% for Veterans with mTBI. Notably, however, the majority of included studies suggest that there are few, if any, significant differences in mental health outcomes for those with mTBI compared to Veteran/military participants without mTBI). Finally, though many individual studies investigated potential moderating factors for mental health outcomes, no clear risk or protective factors were identified; however, studies often reported an association multiple mental health outcomes (e.g., depression, anxiety, and PTSD symptoms were reported to be significantly correlated for those with and without mTBI).

The following table summarizes the evidence on mental health outcomes, which is then followed by detailed results descriptions for specific areas of mental health.

**Table 4. Summary of Evidence for Mental Health Outcomes Associated with mTBI in Veteran and Military Populations**

| Domain (number of studies) | Key Question 1: Estimates of Prevalence and Impairment (number of studies) | Key Question 1: Statistically Significant Deficits Compared to Controls (number of studies) | Key Question 2: Statistically Significant Potential Risk or Protective Factors (number of studies) |
|---|---|---|---|
| PTSD (17) | Yes: Mean scores indicated impairment (4); No: (1)<br><br>Proportion with PTSD = 45% (1) | Mixed (1)<br>No (3) | Yes Protective: Additional injury (1)<br>Yes Risk: Anxiety (1)<br>Yes Risk: Blast exposure (2)<br>Yes Risk: Depression (1)<br>Yes Risk: LOC and/or AOC or PTA (3)<br>Yes Risk: Positive neurological or neuropsychological assessment results (1)<br>Yes Risk: Self-reported cognitive complaints (1)<br>No: Referral to neurology clinic for headaches (1)<br>No: Blast exposure (1) |
| Anxiety (6) | Average anxiety = "moderate-severe" (1)<br><br>Yes: Mean scores indicated impairment (2) | NR | Yes Protective: Additional injury (1)<br>Yes Risk: Depression (1)<br>Yes Risk: LOC and/or PTA (1)<br>Yes Risk: PTSD (2)<br>Yes Risk: Self-reported cognitive complaints (1)<br>No: Blast exposure (1) |
| Depression (8) | Mixed: Mean scores indicated impairment (2) | No (2) | Yes Risk: LOC and/or PTA (1)<br>Yes Risk: PTSD (2)<br>Yes Risk: Self-reported cognitive complaints (1)<br>No: Additional injury (1)<br>No: Blast exposure (1) |
| Substance Use Disorders (2) | Prevalence of alcohol abuse/dependence = 28% (2)<br><br>Prevalence of drug abuse/dependence = 9% (1) | No (2) | Yes Risk: Axis I disorder (1) |
| Suicide (1) | Prevalence of suicidal ideation = 25% (1)<br><br>Prevalence of suicidal intent = 7% (1)<br><br>Prevalence of past suicide attempts = 4% (1) | No (1) | NR |
| Other (6) | Prevalence of Axis I disorder = 50-78% (2)<br><br>Self-reported irritability/ frustration = "moderate-severe" (2) | Yes: Any Axis I disorder (1)<br>No: Any Axis I disorder (1) | Yes Protective: Additional injury (1)<br>Yes Risk: PTSD (2)<br>No: Blast exposure (1) |

*Note.* The impairment summary is based on average scores for groups with mTBI, and does not reflect individual variation in scores which could include some impairment for a certain proportion of participants. "Mixed" results indicate both significant and non-significant results for multiple assessments of the same outcome in a single study.

## PTSD

Key Question 1: There were 17 studies that met inclusion criteria and reported PTSD outcomes (Appendix E, Table 3a).[9-13,16,19-21,25,27,28,31-33,36,38] These studies used the following assessment tools to measure PTSD: Clinician Administered PTSD Scale (CAPS): Total Score and Re-experiencing subscale; PTSD diagnosis; PTSD Checklist - Civilian Version (PCL-C) Total Score, Avoidance subscale, Hyper-Arousal subscale, Re-experiencing subscale, and individual item scores; PTSD Checklist - Military Version (PCL-M); and the PTSD Checklist - Stressor Specific Version (PCL-S). Mean scores on the PCL measures for those with mTBI ranged from 34.6[38] to 61.9,[9] suggesting clinically significant impairment for many with mTBI. Similarly, the one study reporting proportion of patients obtaining scores indicative of clinically significant impairment reported that 45% of individuals with mTBI obtained such scores.[21] Of the studies comparing PTSD in those with mTBI to similar populations without, three reported non-significant differences between groups,[19,21,38] and one provided mixed results.[9]

Key Question 2: One study examined individual items on the PCL-C, and found that all but one (the item asking about disturbing memories) were significantly lower for those who had at least one additional injury.[25] The same study examined the association between PTSD and blast exposure for those with LOC or AOC at the time of injury, describing non-significant findings for all PCL symptom clusters and total scores with the one exception of higher scores on the PCL re-experiencing cluster.[25] Three additional studies examined the association with blast exposure, reporting significantly worse symptoms for those with blast exposure in two of the studies[12,28] and non-significant differences in one study.[16] One study reported significant, positive associations among PTSD, depression, and anxiety symptoms.[20] Two studies reported significantly worse PTSD symptom reports by those with LOC at the time of injury[32] and LOC and/or PTA.[20] One study reported a significant association between PTSD and obtaining positive neurological or neuropsychological test results.[33] One study reported non-significant differences in PTSD between those who were and were not referred to neurology clinics for headache treatment.[31] Finally, one study reported a significant association between self-reported cognitive complaints and PTSD symptoms.[36]

## Anxiety

Key Question 1: We found six primary studies reporting anxiety outcomes including the Hospital Anxiety and Depression Scale (HADS): Anxiety assessment and the NSI: Feeling Anxious item score (Appendix E, Table 3b).[12,13,17,20,25,36] Average self-reported anxiety symptoms were in the moderate-severe range on the NSI and in the clinically significant range on the HADS.[13,36] No studies compared mTBI to non-mTBI populations.

Key Question 2: One study investigating the association of blast exposure with self-reported anxiety resulted in non-significant findings.[12] Four studies reported significantly worse self-reported anxiety for those with PTSD,[12,17] LOC and/or PTA immediate sequelae,[20] self-reported depression,[20] and self-reported slowed thinking, attention deficits, and memory deficits.[36] One study reported that having at least one additional injury was negatively associated with self-reported anxiety.[25]

## Depression

Key Question 1: We found eight primary studies reporting depression outcomes including Beck Depression Inventory 2nd Edition (BDI-II) score, a single-item hopelessness assessment, Hospital Anxiety and Depression Scale (HADS): Depression subscale score, Neurobehavioral Symptom Inventory (NSI): Depression item score, and Structured Clinical Interview for DSM-IV Axis I Disorders (SCID-I): Major Depressive Disorder diagnosis (Appendix E, Table 3c).[9,12,13,17,20,25,36,37] Average self-reported depression severity was in the moderate range on the NSI,[13] though average scores did not fall within the clinically significant range on the HADS.[36] Of the two studies comparing depression symptoms for those with and without mTBI,[9,37] neither reported significantly worse depression symptoms for mTBI participants.

Key Question 2: Two studies investigating the association of blast exposure[12] and additional injury[25] with depression reported non-significant findings. One study investigated presence of LOC and/or PTA[20], two studies investigated PTSD,[12,17] and one study investigated self-reported cognitive problems[36]; all reported that these were statistically significantly associated with worse depression in those with mTBI.

## Substance Use Disorders

Key Question 1: We found only two primary studies reporting substance use outcomes, both using the Structured Clinical Interview for DSM-IV Axis I Disorders (SCID-I) to establish drug or alcohol use/dependence (Appendix E, Table 3d).[9,29] The studies reported that the prevalence of substance use disorders in this population ranged from 9% for drug abuse/dependence[9] to 28% for alcohol abuse/dependence.[9,29] Both studies reported non-significant differences in prevalence compared to controls.

Key Question 2: One of the studies described having another Axis I disorder as significantly associated with increased prevalence of alcohol abuse/dependence.[29]

## Suicide

Key Question 1: We found only one primary study reporting outcomes related to suicide (Appendix E, Table 3e).[9] This study used the following single item assessments of suicide-related outcomes: Suicidal Ideation (Have you had thoughts about death or about killing yourself?), Suicidal Intent (Have you ever intended to commit suicide?), and Past Suicide Attempts (Have you ever attempted suicide?). This single study reported that the prevalence of suicidal ideation in this population was 25%, suicidal intent was 7%, and past suicide attempts was 4%. The authors report non-significant differences when comparing these outcomes to results from non-mTBI controls.

Key Question 2: We did not find any evidence related to this key question.

## Other Mental Health Outcomes

Key Question 1: We found six primary studies reporting other mental health outcomes and summary scores (Appendix E, Table 3f).[9,12,13,18,25,35] The outcomes investigated in these studies included Frontal Systems Behavioral Scale (FrSBe): Apathy pre- to post-injury change and Behavioral Disinhibition pre- to post-injury change subscales, Neurobehavioral Symptom

Inventory (NSI): Affective Cluster, Neurobehavioral Symptom Inventory (NSI): Irritability and Frustration items, Psychiatric Diagnosis, and Structured Clinical Interview for DSM-IV Axis I Disorders (SCID-I): Axis I Disorder diagnosis. The prevalence of Axis I disorder in mTBI populations was reported to range from 50-78% based on two studies, though these same studies report mixed results in terms of whether these prevalence estimates are significantly higher compared to non-mTBI controls.[9,18] Self-reported irritability and frustration were both within the moderate to severe range as assessed by the NSI in one study.[13]

Key Question 2: One study reported a non-significant association between blast exposure and frustration severity.[12] One study reported a significant negative association between having an additional injury and NSI affective cluster, frustration, and irritability scores. [25] Finally, two studies reported that PTSD was significantly associated with poor NSI frustration and irritability item scores[12,18] as well as the NSI affective cluster score.[18]

## FUNCTIONAL/SOCIAL OUTCOME RESULTS

### Summary of Functional/Social Outcome Results

We found 12 studies, all low quality, reporting functional/social outcomes for Veterans or members of the military with mTBI. Due to methodologic limitations as well as small sample size and inadequate reporting of and accounting for time since injury, the strength of evidence for this group of studies is low. One study reported that approximately 20% of Veterans with mTBI experience unemployment. One of two studies comparing participants with mTBI to participants without mTBI found higher unemployment among those with mTBI. Another study found that 26% of those with mTBI had difficulties with interpersonal relationships, though this was not significantly different in comparison to individuals without mTBI. Ten studies examined sleep disturbance: two found an overall prevalence of 13-23% in those with a history of mTBI, and seven found that sleep disturbances, when present, were moderate to severe. One of two studies found that sleep disturbance was more common in those with mTBI compared to those without a history of mTBI. No clear patterns of risk or protective factors emerged from studies examining potential moderators of mTBI history for functional or social outcomes.

The following table summarizes the evidence on functional/social outcomes, which is then followed by detailed results descriptions for each functional/social domain.

**Table 5. Summary of Evidence for Functional/Social Outcomes Associated with mTBI in Veteran and Military Populations**

| Domain (number of studies) | Key Question 1: Estimates of Prevalence and Impairment (number of studies) | Key Question 1: Statistically Significant Deficits Compared to Controls (number of studies) | Key Question 2: Statistically Significant Potential Risk or Protective Factors (number of studies) |
|---|---|---|---|
| Employment (2) | Prevalence of unemployment = 20% (1) | Yes (1) No (1) | No: LOC (1) |
| Sleep (10) | Mixed results related to impairment: Mean self-reported sleep disturbance and fatigue ranged from approximately "mild" to "very severe." (7)<br><br>Prevalence < 4 hours of sleep per night: 13% (1) Prevalence of > 2 hours sleep loss per night: 23% (1) | Yes (1) No (1) | Yes Protective: Additional injury (1) No: Blast exposure (1) Yes Risk: PTSD (2) Yes Risk: Positive neurological or neuropsychological findings (1) Yes Protective: Participation in a headache intervention (1) No: Referral to neurology clinic for headaches(1) |
| Relationships (1) | Prevalence of lack of emotional support = 26% (1) | No (1) | NR |

*Note.* The impairment summary is based on average scores for groups with mTBI, and does not reflect individual variation in scores which could include some impairment for a certain proportion of participants. "Mixed" results indicate both significant and non-significant results for multiple assessments of the same outcome in a single study.

## Employment

Key Question 1: We found only two studies documenting outcomes related to employment status using self-reported unemployment, two or more missed workdays in the past month, difficulty carrying a heavy load in past month, and difficulty performing physical training in past month as indicators of employment outcomes (Appendix E, Table 4a).[9,39] One study described a non-significant comparison to a non-mTBI population, and reported that the rate of unemployment for the mTBI population was 20%.[9] Another study reported that the odds of missing more than 2 days of work ranged from 1.4-1.8, odds of difficulty carrying a heavy load in past month ranged from 2.2-3.0, and odds of difficulty performing physical training in the past month as indicators of employment outcomes ranged from 1.6-1.9 when compared to a non-mTBI reference group.[39]

Key Question 2: One study examined the potential impact of LOC on employment outcomes for Veterans with mTBI, and reported equivalent results across groups for all outcomes assessed. [39]

## Sleep

Key Question 1: We found 10 primary studies that reported sleep outcomes for Veterans and members of the military including the Epworth Sleepiness Scale (ESS); Neurobehavioral Symptom Inventory (NSI): Fatigue and Sleep items; hours per night of sleep; hours per night of sleep lost; and sleep disturbance in the past 30 days.[12,13,15,17,24,25,27,31,33,34] Of the two studies comparing participants with and without mTBI, three out of six sleep outcomes were significantly worse for those with mTBI, and the others were approximately equivalent across groups.[15,24] Only one study reported prevalence of sleep disturbance, estimated at 13% (less than four hours of sleep per night) to 23% (more than 2 hours sleep loss per night) for active duty military personnel within 10 days of injury.[15] Notably, self-reported sleep disturbance and fatigue on the NSI ranged from approximately "mild" (0.86) to approximately "very severe" (3.45) depending on the sub-population with mTBI (e.g., those with and without PTSD), indicating clinically significant impaired sleep for at least some Veterans and members of the military with mTBI.[12,13,17,25,31,33,34]

Key Question 2: One study examining differences between Veterans referred to the neurology clinic for headaches versus those not referred noted non-significant differences between groups on mean NSI sleep item score.[31] Studies examining additional injury,[25] blast exposure,[12] PTSD,[12,17] and positive neurological or neuropsychological findings[33] all suggest that participants with mTBI with these potential risk factors endorse significantly worse sleep disturbance than those without these factors. Similarly, a study investigating a headache intervention described significantly less sleep disturbance endorsed by participants with mTBI who were randomly assigned to the intervention condition compared to the control group of participants with mTBI who were not offered the intervention.[34]

### Social

Key Question 1: We found only one study reporting social outcomes as indicated by lack of emotional support and marital status (Appendix E, Table 4b).[9] This study reported non-significant differences between mTBI compared to non-mTBI participants for both outcomes. The prevalence of lack of emotional support was reported to be 26% for Veterans with mTBI.

Key Question 2: No studies addressed this key question related to social outcomes.

## SERVICE UTILIZATION/COSTS RESULTS

### Summary of Service Utilization/Costs Results

We found seven studies that described service utilization by Veterans with mTBI, and no studies reported costs associated with mTBI. The overall strength of evidence was low because of the small number and methodologic shortcomings of studies. The available literature suggests that there are few differences in service utilization for those with mTBI compared to similar controls, and no significant associations with potential risk or protective factors were identified. The following table summarizes the evidence on service utilization/cost outcomes, which is then followed by a detailed results description of results.

**Table 6. Summary of Evidence for Service Utilization/Costs Associated with mTBI in Veteran and Military Populations**

| Domain (number of studies) | Key Question 1: Estimates of Prevalence and Impairment (number of studies) | Key Question 1: Statistically Significant Deficits Compared to Controls (number of studies) | Key Question 2: Statistically Significant Potential Risk or Protective Factors (number of studies) |
|---|---|---|---|
| Service Utilization (7) | No mean scores indicating impairment (e.g., diagnosis), with the exception of a broad range of results reported for number of prescribed medications. (2)<br><br>Prevalence of current counseling = 4-6%. (1)<br><br>Prevalence of current mental health medications = 4-5%. (1) | No (4) | No: LOC (1) |
| Costs (0) | NR | NR | NR |

*Note.* The impairment summary is based on average scores for groups with mTBI, and does not reflect individual variation in scores which could include some impairment for a certain proportion of participants.

## Service Utilization/Costs

Key Question 1: Table 6 describes the seven primary studies reporting service utilization by Veterans and members of the military including current counseling, current mental health medication, current pain medication, narcotic pain medication, number of medications overall, length of hospital stay, length of intensive care unit stay, and medical utilization as indicated by more than two sick calls within the past month.[10,15,18,21,24,37,39] None of the studies comparing participants with mTBI to those without mTBI[15,18,21,24] or to those with moderate/severe TBI[10] reported statistically significant differences on any service utilization outcomes. One study which did not report a *p*-value, however, reported that participants with mTBI were prescribed an average of 18 medications, compared to a control group without mTBI, who were prescribed an average of five medications.[37] Prevalence of current counseling by those with mTBI was reported to be approximately 4-6% and current mental health medication was 4-5% in two studies of the same population.[15,24]

Key Question 2: One study examined whether or not LOC at the time of injury was related to having two or more sick call visits in the past month, and reported similar odds ratios for mTBI participants with and without LOC.

# SUMMARY AND DISCUSSION

## SUMMARY OF EVIDENCE

We found 31 studies examining the effects of mTBI in Veteran and military populations. In general, though cognitive, physical, and mental health symptoms were commonly reported by Veterans and members of the military following an mTBI, there was little evidence that symptoms were more commonly reported by study participants with mTBI than similar participants without mTBI. However, the evidence base is weakened by inconsistent findings, methodologic shortcomings of many studies, and variation in outcomes considered and outcome measurement approaches. Therefore, conclusions drawn from this body of literature are uncertain, likely to change given additional research in the future, and should be interpreted with caution.

Mental health problems are a serious concern for Veterans and members of the military with mTBI, though the extent to which these outcomes are uniquely related to mTBI versus other deployment-related illnesses are not clear. Posttraumatic stress disorder (PTSD) is one of the most common mental health disorders among Veterans of wartime service, affecting approximately 15% of Veterans of all eras.[40] A recent systematic review estimated the overall prevalence of comorbid TBI and PTSD among OIF/OEF Veterans at 5-7%,[41] and among Veterans with histories of TBI, rates of PTSD range from 33-65%.[41-44] Furthermore, having both PTSD and TBI may adversely affect functionality more than suffering from either disorder alone.[45]

The high prevalence of comorbid PTSD and mTBI are likely related to both event-related factors and neuropsychiatric symptom overlap between disorders.[46] Modern warfare involving multiple deployments and high rates of blast exposure has greatly increased service members' risk of TBI and PTSD.[47] In addition, there is evidence from neuroimaging studies that PTSD and TBI affect similar areas of the brain, including the prefrontal cortex, hippocampus, and amygdala.[47,48] Regardless of etiology, the overlap in the presentation of mTBI and PTSD can be accounted for at least in part by shared symptoms. In particular, core symptoms of both PTSD and postconcussive syndrome include problems with concentration/attention and memory, sleep disturbance, and irritability.[49,50] Moreover, cognitive complaints and objective neurocognitive deficits are common among individuals with PTSD, even in the absence of a history of TBI,[48,51-54] including problems with memory, concentration/attention, and problem-solving.

We found a very limited evidence base examining functional and social outcomes suggesting that one fifth to one quarter of Veterans with mTBI experienced unemployment, sleep disturbance, or lack of emotional support. Whereas more severe levels of TBI are identified immediately post-trauma, cases of mTBI are often unidentified and untreated until after military discharge, at which point Veterans may begin to recognize problems like trouble reintegrating into work or school or difficulties maintaining familial or social relationships. Longitudinal studies have found impairments ranging from difficulty maintaining leisure interests and friendships, to vocational instability, poor life satisfaction, and poor quality of life among individuals who have incurred mTBI.[55,56] Individuals' social and physical environments can either help or hinder recovery of full functional capacity after mTBI. Research has found factors like social support, family adjustment and cohesion, life stressors, and receipt of compensation for disability to be associated with functional outcomes among individuals with mTBI.[57]

The VA will be providing life-long care for a large number of OEF/OIF/OND Veterans who have sustained mTBI. In some cases, the VA will also provide care for the Veterans' informal/ family caregivers.[58] The long-term resource needs of OEF/OIF/OND Veterans are likely substantial; however, these resource needs are possibly related to a variety of factors including comorbid conditions and other consequences of deployment and not uniquely related to having experienced an mTBI. The majority of data on costs and resource utilization of individuals with TBI comes from civilian studies and examines those with moderate-to-severe TBI, for which follow-up care and rehabilitation needs are great and disability is common. Little is known about long-term costs and needs for those with mTBI, particularly military members or Veterans with deployment-related mTBI. Although most outcomes studies of civilians have found that symptoms and sequelae of mTBI resolve within one year after the injury,[59] different contextual factors including mechanism of injury provide only indirect comparisons to Veteran/military outcomes. It is likely that complicating deployment-related factors such as repeat mTBI events or concomitant mental health disorders such as PTSD could result in very different long-term outcomes and resource utilization for this population.

## Findings from Civilian Populations

Though the overall strength of evidence evaluating outcomes following mTBI in Veteran or military populations is low, it is noteworthy that the findings are remarkably consistent with higher quality civilian literature.[59] Both bodies of research suggest that many health consequences resolve within the first few months following injury, if not sooner.

A systematic review of literature in children and adults found objective cognitive deficits associated with mTBI resolve within 2-3 months and the physical consequences of mTBI are likely limited to those which resolve within the first few days following injury.[59] The authors note that though objective cognitive impairment resolves quickly, subjective cognitive complaints may linger for years for some individuals who experience mTBI. They also found that litigation or evaluation for compensation was a risk factor for worse cognitive test performance, a finding echoed by another review.[60]

Other systematic reviews reported similar findings. One review described insufficient and inadequate evidence for any cognitive effects of mTBI greater than 6 months following injury.[61] A meta-analysis of sports-related concussion suggests that though some impairment in memory and global cognitive functioning may be present for individuals with mTBI within a week of injury, these effects are no longer present after 7 days post-injury.[60] These authors also found cognitive deficits were no longer present by 3 months after injury in unselected, consecutive samples.[60]

A systematic review of civilian literature related to functional impairment suggests that there is not a significant impact for children with mTBI, and most functional impairment resolves within a month for adults with mTBI.[59] However, this review also points out that self-reported functional impairment may last longer, up to years, in some instances, particularly when individuals are involved in litigation or compensation related to the mTBI, and when individuals experience the mTBI event as psychologically traumatic.

Pertab and colleagues conducted a re-analysis of studies included in earlier meta-analyses. This group of authors suggests that time since injury and the use of different cognitive assessment tools may have a potentially moderating effect on cognitive outcomes.[62] The authors describe a range in summary effect sizes based on cognitive domain and time since injury, suggesting the possibility that some subgroups of those with mTBI may experience some objective cognitive deficits for a limited period of time following injury.

Of note, the WHO Collaborating Centre for Neurotrauma Prevention, Management and Rehabilitation Task Force has recently completed an updated systematic review examining the effects of mTBI in civilian populations. Results are likely to be reported within the next year and should further add to our understanding.

Even though the strength of evidence in civilian populations is higher, there is not enough information in that body of literature either to identify how factors such as time since injury, mechanism of injury, or number of mTBIs influence long-term outcomes.

## Use of Imaging and Biomarkers in mTBI Research

Although beyond the scope of this review, since imaging and biomarker technologies are a rapidly evolving area of research of interest to stakeholders, we will briefly summarize recent relevant research here.

Although biomarkers are increasingly being used as prognostic tools among those with moderate or severe TBI, research among those with less severe injuries has been limited.[63] Efforts are focused on evaluating serum and cerebral spinal fluid during different stages of the brain injury cascade (e.g., inflammation, neuronal injury).[64] As no single biomarker with discriminative characteristics has been indentified, Sharma and Laskowitz (2012) suggest that combining biomarkers may increase sensitivity and specificity.[64] For further information regarding biomarkers and mTBI see Jeter et al. (2012), and Sharma and Laskowitz (2012).[64,65]

Recent interest has emerged regarding the possibility that returning military personnel with a history of TBI are at risk for developing chronic traumatic encephalopathy (CTE).[66] CTE refers to persistent cognitive and neuropsychiatric symptoms (e.g., executive dysfunction, memory impairment, depression, poor impulse control, and dementia) secondary to chronic neurodegeneration thought to be caused at least in part by multiple TBIs.[67] At present, CTE can only be identified by direct tissue examination; as such, full autopsies and immunohistochemical brain analyses are necessary for definitive diagnosis. Despite much speculation regarding blast exposed individuals being at risk for CTE, limited data currently exists in support of this relationship. Current efforts pertaining to increasing understanding regarding CTE include: creating clinical diagnostic criteria, identifying objective biomarkers, and increasing understanding regarding additional risk factors and underlying mechanisms.[68]

Recent literature reviews of neuroimaging in mTBI including DTI, functional,[69] and metabolic imaging,[70] have examined the association of imaging findings with neuropathology.[71] Although brain changes resulting from mTBI are often not discernible with conventional clinical structural CT and MRI, there is a growing body of evidence that they are more readily detectible with advanced research imaging technologies, particularly DTI,[72] which measures the functional integrity of white matter interconnections within the brain. A rapidly growing body of DTI investigation indicates that DTI is more sensitive to white matter injury than conventional MRI and CT, with DTI consistently detecting more abnormalities than conventional CT or MRI across multiple mTBI studies. As would be expected from the animal model and neurocognitive assessment literature,[71] acute and subacute structural and functional imaging changes are demonstrated. However, abnormalities have also been demonstrated at chronic stages, suggesting that some patients experience long-term brain changes as well. The most common abnormalities have been shown for long association pathways including the corticospinal tract, corpus callosum, corona radiata, internal capsule, uncinate fasciculus, and the superior longitudinal fasciculus. Further, in some studies, DTI abnormalities correlate with cognitive performance in patients with mTBI, with general aggregate DTI abnormality correlated with executive function, memory, and cognitive processing speed. Locally specific structure-function relationships have sometimes been observed in mTBI, with damage to frontal white matter associated with executive function and attentional performance, and temporal tract changes associated with decreases in memory performance. Some more recent imaging studies support the notion of persistent postconcussive symptoms (PCS), with observable pathophysiological findings correlated with PCS. Supportive of these DTI findings, many fMRI studies found activation differences between individuals with mTBI and individuals in the control group during cognitive and behavioral tasks consistent with DTI findings, although many studies failed to show associated significant differences in task performance.[69] The various metabolic imaging techniques are less well investigated in mTBI, but initial results suggest that these techniques show promise as investigative and diagnostic tools.[70]

Although rapidly growing, there remain several limitations for mTBI neuroimaging research. It is largely made up of cross-sectional studies with small samples, and there is a great deal of method and design variability with respect to such factors as time period of scanning post-injury, brain regions examined, magnet strength, non-imaging outcome variables, and methods of analyses, resulting in differences across studies in both anatomical location of observed brain alterations and the nature of these alterations. Despite considerable consistency in its main findings, this body of research is still relatively new and there remain as-yet unresolved discrepancies. For instance, some DTI studies show increased fractional anisotropy (FA), while others show decreased FA. Also, many fMRI studies failed to show associated significant differences in task performance associated with significant task-related activation differences between patients and control participants.[69] Imaging studies nonetheless are consistent in providing evidence of small and subtle brain injuries in mTBI that are often, although not always, associated with symptoms and cognitive performance. This evidence would not be possible if conventional MRI and CT scans alone were used to establish and characterize brain injury; it requires more advanced and sophisticated imaging methods such as DTI and fMRI that are sensitive to the effects of diffuse axonal injury and altered metabolic function to delineate these abnormalities.

## Clinical Considerations

The best available evidence, which is of low quality, suggests that many symptoms that patients ascribe to mTBI may be related to comorbid mental or physical health concerns, or to other factors such as readjustment to civilian life following deployment or injury beliefs and perceptions.[73] Difficulties related to post-deployment adjustment underscores the need to engage recently returned Veterans and members of the military quickly in efforts to identify physical and mental health problems and provide appropriate re-integration services. Patients should be encouraged to engage in treatment for these comorbid concerns with the best available evidence-based treatments (e.g., evidence-based psychotherapy to treat PTSD).

Administrators setting policy for treatment of military-related mTBI should be cautioned to treat the available evidence as limited and subject to change depending on findings from future, more methodologically rigorous studies. Policy based on the best available evidence should likely encourage the treatment of comorbid conditions that commonly occur for Veterans and members of the military who have experienced deployment (e.g., treatment for PTSD, substance use disorders, headaches, sleep disorders, and other post-deployment concerns).

Given the lack of large, good-quality observational studies with adequate follow-up it is very difficult to estimate the long-term cognitive effects of mTBI. However, the current evidence base suggests that cognitive deficits are not common, particularly more than three months after injury. Therefore, should individuals with mTBI continue to experience ongoing cognitive deficits following first-line treatment for co-occurring symptoms and disorders such as PTSD, further testing such as neuropsychological or neurological evaluations or imaging might be warranted.

## LIMITATIONS AND RECOMMENDATIONS FOR FUTURE RESEARCH

The available literature reporting consequences of mTBI in Veteran and military populations is based on low quality observational studies and provides low strength evidence for the associations synthesized in this systematic review. Notably, not all outcomes of potential interest to stakeholders were found in the literature base (e.g., costs). There is insufficient data to determine the presence or absence of an effect for these outcomes, and further research is warranted.

One of the major limitations of this literature is the inadequate reporting of and accounting for time since injury among Veterans and military members, and therefore it is not possible to construct an accurate picture of mTBI consequences over time for this population. This body of literature is also likely subject to participant recall bias due to the cross-sectional, retrospective nature of almost all included studies. Participants are likely unable to accurately recall symptoms and timeframes so long after one (or more) mTBI events. Future research should take advantage of available VA and DoD databases that have time since injury information and include this variable in the analysis of mTBI consequences on an individual participant level. Similarly, such databases should be used to examine the possible effect of multiple mTBI events as this is a common occurrence for many individuals who were part of OEF/OIF conflicts. Additionally, a large prospective cohort study would be better able to identify factors associated with outcomes in mTBI populations.

A related limitation of the body of literature relates to how data is presented in included studies. Very few studies reported the actual prevalence of symptoms or conditions; most studies simply reported mean scores for the entire study group. This latter approach can provide useful information for determining whether there is a unique contribution of mTBI versus outcomes being affected by more general deployment or combat exposure factors. However, a lack of prevalence estimates limits an accurate description of the population, particularly when a goal of stakeholders is to estimate numbers of Veterans who will be affected by specific outcomes and utilize related treatment services. Future research should not only report mean scores for subgroups, but also report proportions of individuals with clinically significant impairment for each outcome. This recommendation is particularly relevant to the body of research on cognitive outcomes, as the vast majority of this literature describes differences based on means rather than reporting the proportion of individuals who obtain scores indicating impaired functioning. For cognitive outcomes in particular, impairment is ideally determined not only by standardized scores within a certain range, but also by comparison to pre-injury (baseline) functioning. Studies should report this intra-individual change as part of any cognitive findings so that accurate estimates of mTBI-related cognitive impairment are reported.

Few studies presented data on all outcomes of interest to the stakeholders of this review, and few studies reported their outcome reporting rationale. Most studies relied on clinical datasets, which are generally not maintained for research purposes, rather than research databases or registries. The use of these datasets can be efficient relative to primary data collection but typically do not contain all variables of interest in a given scientific inquiry. It is likely that many studies only included outcomes of relevance to the authors' particular study questions, though it is impossible to know whether some studies did not report outcomes given a lack of association with mTBI. There is a pressing need for large cohort studies of Veterans with and without mTBI that prospectively collect data on all risk and protective factors, and all outcomes of interest. Such studies would be relatively costly but would result in higher-quality evidence on which more definitive conclusions could be based.

Although a strength of this review was that many of the included studies relied on well-validated measures commonly used with Veteran/military populations, many of the clinical outcomes relied solely on self-reported outcomes, often obtained from single questionnaire items. Self-report data is often the only way to assess certain outcomes such as pain. However, some notable results from this review and a review of the civilian literature[59] suggest that self-reported deficits are more likely to be reported by individuals with mTBI. Assessment for mTBI is often associated with potential financial compensation, which in turn has been commonly associated with worse outcomes. Because participants are not often blinded to study hypotheses, self-reported outcomes should be interpreted with greater caution than objective findings evaluated by blinded outcome assessors. Thus, future research should consider using objective and validated assessments, blinded outcome assessors, patient blinding to study hypotheses, and accounting for compensation factors whenever possible in order to reduce bias associated with outcome assessment.

Additionally, future research should employ commonly used outcome assessment tools in order to facilitate the combination of results across studies for meta-analytic purposes. One of the limitations of this body of literature was the wide variety of tools used to assess each outcome. Though we reported statistically significant results from included studies, it is possible that combining studies mathematically would increase power, and effects could be detected in aggregate which were not apparent at the individual study level. In the case of this review, diversity in outcome assessment tools precluded mathematical combination of results.[74]

A final strength of this review was the use of clear criteria for defining mTBI. However, because the majority of studies did not assess or report imaging results, and those that did were inconsistent in their inclusion of participants with positive imaging results, we were not able to apply exclusion criteria based on positive imaging as is recommended by the VA/DoD definition of mTBI. Additionally, because of our reliance on stringent definitional criteria, we excluded many studies that purported to study mTBI populations, but did not meet the criteria for this report. The scope of this report focused explicitly on OEF/OIF/OND Veterans and members of the military meeting VA/DoD mTBI criteria; consequently, this report provides a narrow window of information on mTBI and should not be viewed as comprehensive. Findings from other systematic reviews on mTBI in civilian populations should be considered for a more complete understanding of mTBI consequences. Future primary research should clearly report criteria used to define mTBI, including assessment and reporting of imaging results. Future research should investigate the possible impact of number of mTBI events, as many studies noted that Veterans experienced multiple mTBIs, though few examined this variable as a possible moderator of outcomes. Additionally, future reviews should consider examination of differences in outcomes based on definitional criteria for mTBI, as it is possible that less stringent criteria could be associated with different results.

## CONCLUSIONS

Overall, given the low strength of evidence, it is difficult to draw firm conclusions about the effects of mTBI in Veteran and military populations. The literature reviewed here is relatively consistent with findings from the more methodologically rigorous, prospective, longitudinal studies conducted in civilian populations. Both bodies of literature suggest that though some negative outcomes occur for a significant portion of individuals who have mTBI, most objective results (e.g., objective cognitive test results) are not significantly different from control participants, and deficits that are present shortly following injury most often resolve within days to months. The literature on Veterans and members of the military suggests that many have physical and mental health symptoms, but it is not clear that those with mTBI experience more or higher severity symptoms than those without mTBI suggesting that outcomes may be influenced by other deployment-related conditions such as PTSD. The studies included in this report were low quality, cross sectional studies which did not provide consistent evidence for potential moderators of mTBI outcomes.

# REFERENCES

1.    Hoge CW, Goldberg HM, Castro CA. Care of war veterans with mild traumatic brain injury--flawed perspectives. *N Engl J Med.* Apr 16 2009;360(16):1588-1591.

2.    Ruff R. Two decades of advances in understanding of mild traumatic brain injury. *J Head Trauma Rehabil.* Jan-Feb 2005;20(1):5-18.

3.    Wood RL. Understanding the 'miserable minority': a diasthesis-stress paradigm for post-concussional syndrome. *Brain Inj.* 2004;18(11):1135-1153.

4.    Cancelliere C, Cassidy JD, Côté P, et al. Protocol for a systematic review of prognosis after mild traumatic brain injury: an update of the WHO Collaborating Centre Task Force findings. *Systematic Reviews.* 2012;1:17.

5.    Lin H, Ling S, Liu Z, Zhong X, Chen W. Preventive scleral buckling and silicone oil tamponade are important for posttraumatic endophthalmitis successfully managed with vitrectomy. *Ophthalmologica.* 2011;226(4):214-219.

6.    Goldman SM, Tanner CM, Oakes D, Bhudhikanok GS, Gupta A, Langston JW. Head injury and Parkinson's disease risk in twins. *Ann Neurol.* Jul 2006;60(1):65-72.

7.    Wells GA, Shea B, O'Connell D, et al. Newcastle Ottawa scales 2009; http://www.ohri. ca/programs/clinical_epidemiology/oxford.asp.

8.    Guyatt G, Oxman AD, Akl EA, et al. GRADE guidelines: 1. Introduction-GRADE evidence profiles and summary of findings tables. *J Clin Epidemiol.* Apr 2011;64(4):383-394.

9.    Barnes SM, Walter KH, Chard KM. Does a history of mild traumatic brain injury increase suicide risk in veterans with PTSD? *Rehabil Psychol.* Feb 2012;57(1):18-26.

10.   Belanger HG, Kretzmer T, Vanderploeg RD, French LM. Symptom complaints following combat-related traumatic brain injury: relationship to traumatic brain injury severity and posttraumatic stress disorder. *J Int Neuropsychol Soc.* Jan 2010;16(1):194-199.

11.   Belanger HG, Kretzmer T, Yoash-Gantz R, Pickett T, Tupler LA. Cognitive sequelae of blast-related versus other mechanisms of brain trauma. *J Int Neuropsychol Soc.* Jan 2009;15(1):1-8.

12.   Belanger HG, Proctor-Weber Z, Kretzmer T, Kim M, French LM, Vanderploeg RD. Symptom complaints following reports of blast versus non-blast mild TBI: does mechanism of injury matter? *Clin Neuropsychol.* Jul 2011;25(5):702-715.

13.   Benge JF, Pastorek NJ, Thornton GM. Postconcussive symptoms in OEF-OIF veterans: factor structure and impact of posttraumatic stress. *Rehabil Psychol.* Aug 2009;54(3):270-278.

14.    Coldren RL, Kelly MP, Parish RV, Dretsch M, Russell ML. Evaluation of the Military Acute Concussion Evaluation for use in combat operations more than 12 hours after injury. *Mil Med.* Jul 2010;175(7):477-481.

15.    Coldren RL, Russell ML, Parish RV, Dretsch M, Kelly MP. The ANAM lacks utility as a diagnostic or screening tool for concussion more than 10 days following injury. *Mil Med.* Feb 2012;177(2):179-183.

16.    Cooper DB, Chau PM, Armistead-Jehle P, Vanderploeg RD, Bowles AO. Relationship between mechanism of injury and neurocognitive functioning in OEF/OIF service members with mild traumatic brain injuries. *Mil Med.* 2012;177(10):1157-1160.

17.    Cooper DB, Kennedy JE, Cullen MA, Critchfield E, Amador RR, Bowles AO. Association between combat stress and post-concussive symptom reporting in OEF/OIF service members with mild traumatic brain injuries. *Brain Inj.* 2011;25(1):1-7.

18.    Cooper DB, Mercado-Couch JM, Critchfield E, et al. Factors influencing cognitive functioning following mild traumatic brain injury in OIF/OEF burn patients. *NeuroRehabilitation.* 2010;26(3):233-238.

19.    Cooper DB, Nelson L, Armistead-Jehle P, Bowles AO. Utility of the mild brain injury atypical symptoms scale as a screening measure for symptom over-reporting in operation enduring freedom/operation iraqi freedom service members with post-concussive complaints. *Arch Clin Neuropsychol.* Dec 2011;26(8):718-727.

20.    Drag LL, Spencer RJ, Walker SJ, Pangilinan PH, Bieliauskas LA. The Contributions of Self-reported Injury Characteristics and Psychiatric Symptoms to Cognitive Functioning in OEF/OIF Veterans with Mild Traumatic Brain Injury. *J Int Neuropsychol Soc.* May 2012;18(3):576-584.

21.    Gaylord KM, Cooper DB, Mercado JM, Kennedy JE, Yoder LH, Holcomb JB. Incidence of posttraumatic stress disorder and mild traumatic brain injury in burned service members: preliminary report. *J Trauma.* Feb 2008;64(2 Suppl):S200-205; discussion S205-206.

22.    Gordon SN, Fitzpatrick PJ, Hilsabeck RC. No effect of PTSD and other psychiatric disorders on cognitive functioning in veterans with mild TBI. *Clin Neuropsychol.* Apr 2011;25(3):337-347.

23.    Gottshall K, Drake A, Gray N, McDonald E, Hoffer ME. Objective vestibular tests as outcome measures in head injury patients. *Laryngoscope.* Oct 2003;113(10):1746-1750.

24.    Kelly MP, Coldren RL, Parish RV, Dretsch MN, Russell ML. Assessment of acute concussion in the combat environment. *Arch Clin Neuropsychol.* Jun 2012;27(4):375-388.

25.    Kennedy JE, Cullen MA, Amador RR, Huey JC, Leal FO. Symptoms in military service members after blast mTBI with and without associated injuries. *NeuroRehabilitation.* 2010;26(3):191-197.

26.    Kennedy JE, Leal FO, Lewis JD, Cullen MA, Amador RR. Posttraumatic stress
       symptoms in OIF/OEF service members with blast-related and non-blast-related mild
       TBI. *NeuroRehabilitation.* 2010;26(3):223-231.

27.    Lew HL, Pogoda TK, Hsu P-T, et al. Impact of the "polytrauma clinical triad" on sleep
       disturbance in a department of veterans affairs outpatient rehabilitation setting. *Am J Phys
       Med Rehabil.* Jun 2010;89(6):437-445.

28.    Lippa SM, Pastorek NJ, Benge JF, Thornton GM. Postconcussive symptoms after blast
       and nonblast-related mild traumatic brain injuries in Afghanistan and Iraq war veterans. *J
       Int Neuropsychol Soc.* Sep 2010;16(5):856-866.

29.    Nelson WN, Hoelzle JB, Doane BM, et al. Neuropsychological Outcomes of U.S.
       Veterans with Report of Remote Blast-Related Concussion and Current Psychopathology.
       *J Int Neuropsychol Soc.* 2012;18:1-11.

30.    Nelson NW, Hoelzle JB, McGuire KA, Ferrier-Auerbach AG, Charlesworth MJ,
       Sponheim SR. Evaluation context impacts neuropsychological performance of OEF/
       OIF veterans with reported combat-related concussion. *Arch Clin Neuropsychol.* Dec
       2010;25(8):713-723.

31.    Patil VK, St Andre JR, Crisan E, et al. Prevalence and treatment of headaches in veterans
       with mild traumatic brain injury. *Headache.* Jul-Aug 2011;51(7):1112-1121.

32.    Ruff RL, Riechers RG, 2nd, Wang X-F, Piero T, Ruff SS. A case-control study examining
       whether neurological deficits and PTSD in combat veterans are related to episodes of
       mild TBI. *BMJ Open.* 2012;2(2):e000312.

33.    Ruff RL, Ruff SS, Wang X-F. Headaches among Operation Iraqi Freedom/Operation
       Enduring Freedom veterans with mild traumatic brain injury associated with exposures to
       explosions. *J Rehabil Res Dev.* 2008;45(7):941-952.

34.    Ruff RL, Ruff SS, Wang X-F. Improving sleep: initial headache treatment in OIF/
       OEF veterans with blast-induced mild traumatic brain injury. *J Rehabil Res Dev.*
       2009;46(9):1071-1084.

35.    Schiehser DM, Delis DC, Filoteo JV, et al. Are self-reported symptoms of executive
       dysfunction associated with objective executive function performance following mild to
       moderate traumatic brain injury? *J Clin Exp Neuropsychol.* Jul 2011;33(6):704-714.

36.    Spencer RJ, Drag LL, Walker SJ, Bieliauskas LA. Self-reported cognitive symptoms
       following mild traumatic brain injury are poorly associated with neuropsychological
       performance in OIF/OEF veterans. *J Rehabil Res Dev.* 2010;47(6):521-530.

37.    Swick D, Honzel N, Larsen J, Ashley V, Justus T. Impaired response inhibition in
       veterans with post-traumatic stress disorder and mild traumatic brain injury. *J Int
       Neuropsychol Soc.* Sep 2012;18(5):917-926.

38.   Theeler BJ, Erickson JC. Mild head trauma and chronic headaches in returning US soldiers. *Headache.* Apr 2009;49(4):529-534.

39.   Toblin RL, Riviere LA, Thomas JL, Adler AB, Kok BC, Hoge CW. Grief and physical health outcomes in U.S. soldiers returning from combat. *J Affect Disord.* Feb 2012;136(3):469-475.

40.   Wagner A, Jakupcak M. Combat-related stress reactions among U.S. veterans of wartime service. In: Matthews JHLMD, ed. *The Oxford Handbook of Military Psychology.* New York: Oxford University Press; 2012:15-28.

41.   Carlson KF, Kehle SM, Meis LA, et al. Prevalence, assessment, and treatment of mild traumatic brain injury and posttraumatic stress disorder: a systematic review of the evidence. *J Head Trauma Rehabil.* Mar-Apr 2011;26(2):103-115.

42.   Cohen B, Gima K, Bertenthal D, Kim S, Marmar C, Seal K. Mental Health Diagnoses and Utilization of VA Non-Mental Health Medical Services Among Returning Iraq and Afghanistan Veterans. *J Gen Intern Med.* 2010;25(1):18-24.

43.   Lew HL, Otis JD, Tun C, Kerns RD, Clark ME, Cifu DX. Prevalence of chronic pain, posttraumatic stress disorder, and persistent postconcussive symptoms in OIF/OEF veterans: polytrauma clinical triad. *J Rehabil Res Dev.* 2009;46(6):697-702.

44.   Pietrzak RH, Johnson DC, Goldstein MB, Malley JC, Southwick SM. Posttraumatic stress disorder mediates the relationship between mild traumatic brain injury and health and psychosocial functioning in veterans of Operations Enduring Freedom and Iraqi Freedom. *J Nerv Ment Dis.* Oct 2009;197(10):748-753.

45.   Uomoto JM, Williams RM, Randa LA. Neurobehavioral consequences of combat-related blast injury and polytrauma. *Ashley, Mark J [Ed].* 2010:63-95.

46.   Vasterling JJ, Bryant RA, Keane TM. Understanding the interface of traumatic stress and mild traumatic brain injury: Background and conceptual framework. *Vasterling, Jennifer J [Ed].* 2012:3-11.

47.   Bogdanova Y, Verfaellie M. Cognitive sequelae of blast-induced traumatic brain injury: recovery and rehabilitation. *Neuropsychol Rev.* Mar 2012;22(1):4-20.

48.   Dolan S, Martindale S, Robinson J, et al. Neuropsychological sequelae of PTSD and TBI following war deployment among OEF/OIF veterans. *Neuropsychol Rev.* Mar 2012;22(1):21-34.

49.   APA APA. *Diagnostic and statistical manual of mental disorders (Revised 4th ed.).* Washington, DC2000.

50.   Ruff R, Grant I. Postconcussional disorder: Background to DSM-IV and future considerations. In: Roberts NRVRJ, ed. *Evaluation and treatment of mild traumatic brain injury.* Mahwah,: Lawrence Erlbaum Associates, Inc; 1999.

51.    Brewin CR, Kleiner JS, Vasterling JJ, Field AP. Memory for emotionally neutral
       information in posttraumatic stress disorder: A meta-analytic investigation. *Journal of
       Abnormal Psychology.* Aug 2007;116(3):448-463.

52.    Leskin LP, White PM. Attentional networks reveal executive function deficits in
       posttraumatic stress disorder. *Neuropsychology.* May 2007;21(3):275-284.

53.    Vasterling JJ, Brailey K, Constans JI, Sutker PB. Attention and memory dysfunction in
       posttraumatic stress disorder. *Neuropsychology.* Jan 1998;12(1):125-133.

54.    Vasterling JJ, Proctor SP. Understanding the neuropsychological consequences of
       deployment stress: a public health framework. *J Int Neuropsychol Soc.* Jan 2011;17(1):1-
       6.

55.    High WMJ, Sander AM, Struchen MA, Hart KA. *Rehabilitation for Traumatic Brain
       Injury.* New York, NY: Oxford University Press; 2005.

56.    Crooks CY, Zumsteg JM, Bell KR. Traumatic Brain Injury: A Review of Practice
       Management and Recent Advances. *Physical medicine and rehabilitation clinics of North
       America.* 2007;18(4):681-710.

57.    McCrea M. Functional Outcome after mTBI. In: Series OW, ed. *Mild Traumatic Brain
       Injury and Postconcussion Syndrome: The New Evidence Base for Diagnosis and
       Treatment.* New York, NY: Oxford University Press; 2008.

58.    Public Law -. Caregivers and Veterans Omnibus Health Services Act of 2010 United
       States Government Printing Office; 2010.

59.    Carroll LJ, Cassidy JD, Peloso PM, et al. Prognosis for mild traumatic brain injury:
       results of the who collaborating centre task force on mild traumatic brain injury. *J
       Rehabil Med.* 2004;36(Supplement 43):84-105.

60.    Belanger HG, Vanderploeg RD. The neuropsychological impact of sports-related
       concussion: a meta-analysis. *J Int Neuropsychol Soc.* Jul 2005;11(4):345-357.

61.    Dikmen SS, Corrigan JD, Levin HS, Machamer J, Stiers W, Weisskopf MG. Cognitive
       outcome following traumatic brain injury. *J Head Trauma Rehabil.* Nov-Dec
       2009;24(6):430-438.

62.    Pertab JL, James KM, Bigler ED. Limitations of mild traumatic brain injury meta-
       analyses. *Brain Inj.* 2009;23(6):498-508.

63.    Metting Z, Wilczak N, Rodiger LA, Schaaf JM, van der Naalt J. GFAP and S100B in the
       acute phase of mild traumatic brain injury. *Neurology.* May 1 2012;78(18):1428-1433.

64.    Sharma R, Laskowitz DT. Biomarkers in traumatic brain injury. *Curr Neurol Neurosci
       Rep.* Oct 2012;12(5):560-569.

65.     Jeter CB, Hergenroeder GW, Hylin MJ, Redell JB, Moore AN, Dash PK. Biomarkers for the diagnosis and prognosis of mild traumatic brain injury/concussion. *J Neurotrauma.* 2012;Oct 12 (Epub ahead of print).

66.     Goldstein LE, Fisher AM, Tagge CA. Chronic traumatic encephalopathy in blast-exposed military veterans and a blast neurotrauma mouse model. *Sci Transl Med.* 2012;4(134):134ra160.

67.     Omalu B, I., Bailes J, Hammers JL, Fitzsimmons RP. Chronic Traumatic Encephalopathy, Suicides and Parasuicides in Professional American Athletes: The Role of the Forensic Pathologist. *American Journal of Forensic Medicine & Pathology June.* 2010;31(2):130-132.

68.     Baugh CM, Stamm JM, Riley DO, et al. Chronic traumatic encephalopathy: neurodegeneration following repetitive concussive and subconcussive brain trauma. *Brain imaging behav.* Jun 2012;6(2):244-254.

69.     McDonald BC, Saykin AJ, McAllister TW. Functional MRI of mild traumatic brain injury (mTBI): progress and perspectives from the first decade of studies. *Brain imaging behav.* Jun 2012;6(2):193-207.

70.     Lin AP, Liao HJ, Merugumala SK, Prabhu SP, Meehan WP, 3rd, Ross BD. Metabolic imaging of mild traumatic brain injury. *Brain imaging behav.* Jun 2012;6(2):208-223.

71.     Bigler ED, Maxwell WL. Neuropathology of mild traumatic brain injury: relationship to neuroimaging findings. *Brain imaging behav.* Jun 2012;6(2):108-136.

72.     Shenton M, Hamoda H, Schneiderman J, et al. A review of magnetic resonance imaging and diffusion tensor imaging findings in mild traumatic brain injury. *Brain Imaging and Behavior.* Jun 2012;6(2):137-192.

73.     Whittaker R, Kemp S, House A. Illness perceptions and outcome in mild head injury: a longitudinal study. *J Neurol Neurosurg Psychiatry.* 2007;78(6):644-646.

74.     Wilde EA, Whiteneck GG, Bogner J, et al. Recommendations for the Use of Common Outcome Measures in Traumatic Brain Injury Research. *Archives of physical medicine and rehabilitation.* 2010;91(11):1650-1660.e1617.

75.     Morissette SB, Woodward M, Kimbrel NA, et al. Deployment-related TBI, persistent postconcussive symptoms, PTSD, and depression in OEF/OIF veterans. *Rehabil Psychol.* Nov 2011;56(4):340-350.

# APPENDIX A. SEARCH STRATEGIES

Database: Ovid MEDLINE(R) and Ovid OLDMEDLINE(R) <1946 to September Week 3 2012>, Ovid MEDLINE(R) In-Process & Other Non-Indexed Citations <October 02, 2012>

Search Strategy:

--------------------------------------------------------------------------------

| | |
|---|---|
| 1 | exp Brain edema/ (11605) |
| 2 | exp cerebrovascular trauma/ (4960) |
| 3 | exp craniocerebral trauma/ (113847) |
| 4 | exp coma/ (17150) |
| 5 | exp glasgow outcome scale/ (1042) |
| 6 | exp glasgow coma scale/ (6068) |
| 7 | ((brain* or capitis or cerebr* or crani* or hemispher* or inter-crani* or intra-crani* or skull*) adj4 (contusion* or damag* or fractur* or injur* or trauma* or wound*)).ab,ti. (77042) |
| 8 | ((brain or crani* or cerebr* or head or inter-cran* or intra-cran*) adj4 (bleed* or haematoma* or haemorrhag* or hematoma* or hemorrhag* or pressure)).ti,ab. (23995) |
| 9 | (Glasgow adj (coma or outcome) adj (scale* or score*)).ab,ti. (7439) |
| 10 | 'Rancho Los Amigos Scale'.ti,ab. (31) |
| 11 | diffuse axonal injur*.ti,ab. (755) |
| 12 | ((brain or cerebral or intracranial) adj3 (edema or oedema or swell*)).ab,ti. (11389) |
| 13 | ((coma* or concuss* or unconscious* or 'persistent vegetative state') adj2 (damag* or fractur* or injur* or trauma* or wound*)).ti,ab. (1686) |
| 14 | (mtbi or "mild trauma* injur*").tw. or "minor trauma* injur*".mp. (639) |
| 15 | 1 or 2 or 3 or 4 or 5 or 6 or 7 or 8 or 9 or 10 or 11 or 12 or 13 or 14 (209513) |
| 16 | exp cohort studies/ (1212058) |
| 17 | exp prognosis/ (967036) |
| 18 | exp morbidity/ (328065) |
| 19 | exp mortality/ (255922) |
| 20 | exp survival analysis/ (158174) |
| 21 | exp models, statistical/ (230839) |
| 22 | prognos*.tw. (324957) |
| 23 | course*.tw. (428896) |
| 24 | diagnosed.tw. (303319) |
| 25 | cohort*.tw. (221535) |
| 26 | death.tw. (417341) |
| 27 | predict*.tw. (808663) |
| 28 | 16 or 17 or 18 or 19 or 20 or 21 or 22 or 23 or 24 or 25 or 26 or 27 (3743025) |
| 29 | diagnosed.tw. (303319) |
| 30 | cohort:.mp. (281196) |
| 31 | (predictor: or death).tw. (578864) |
| 32 | exp models, statistical/ (230839) |
| 33 | prognosis/ (327999) |

34    29 or 30 or 31 or 32 or 33 (1494750)

35    28 or 34 (3743144)

36    15 and 35 (67135)

37    exp rehabilitation, vocational/ (8852)

38    exp employment/ (49891)

39    exp work/ (12406)

40    sick leave/ (3365)

41    absenteeism/ (6861)

42    exp occupational health/ (23070)

43    exp occupational medicine/ (21574)

44    exp disabled persons/ (43220)

45    "recovery of function"/ (25824)

46    exp human activities/ (291441)

47    exp self care/ (36358)

48    activities of daily living.tw. (13206)

49    (dressing or feeding or eating or toilet$ or bathing or mobil$ or driving or public transport$).tw. (409253)

50    ((daily or domestic or house or home) adj5 (activit$ or task$ or skill$ or chore$)).tw. (34321)

51    ("work status" or "work capacity").tw. (4948)

52    (unemployment or re-employment or underemployment or "job retention").ti,ab. (6217)

53    (return* adj2 school).tw. (428)

54    37 or 38 or 39 or 40 or 41 or 42 or 43 or 44 or 45 or 46 or 47 or 48 or 49 or 50 or 51 or 52 or 53 (884984)

55    15 and 54 (12268)

56    exp dementia/ (109281)

57    Delirium/ or exp Delirium, Dementia, Amnestic, Cognitive Disorders/ (165121)

58    dement*.mp. or alzheimer*.tw. (137451)

59    exp Parkinsonian Disorders/ (53442)

60    parkinson*.tw. (67897)

61    56 or 57 or 58 or 59 or 60 (263117)

62    15 and 61 (10666)

63    36 or 55 or 62 (80547)

64    animals/ not (humans/ and animals/) (3693774)

65    63 not 64 (72473)

66    limit 65 to (danish or english or french or norwegian or spanish or swedish) (62699)

67    limit 66 to yr="2001 -Current" (36478)

68    exp "Outcome Assessment (Health Care)"/ (605282)

69    (intervention* adj3 stud*).tw. (23915)

70    68 or 69 (626005)

71    15 and 70 (12781)

72    71 not 64 (12055)

73    limit 72 to (yr="2001 -Current" and (danish or english or french or norwegian or swedish)) (8537)

74    67 or 73 (36658)

75   randomized controlled trial.pt. (337763)
76   Randomized controlled trial/ (337763)
77   Randomized Controlled Trials as Topic/ (83241)
78   Double-Blind Method/ (117191)
79   clinical trial.pt. (474276)
80   "double blind:".mp. (143695)
81   placebos/ (31353)
82   placebo:.mp. (158293)
83   random:.mp. (788646)
84   75 or 76 or 77 or 78 or 79 or 80 or 81 or 82 or 83 (1069355)
85   15 and 84 (10248)
86   review/ (1739065)
87   (medline or medlars or pubmed or grateful med or CINAHL or scisearch or psychinfo
     or psycinfo or psychlit or psyclit or handsearch* or hand search* or manual* search* or
     electronic database* or bibliographic database* or embase or lilacs or scopus or web of
     science).mp. (74569)
88   86 and 87 (48085)
89   meta-analysis.mp. (59484)
90   meta-analysis as topic/ (12450)
91   meta-analysis/ (36480)
92   systematic review*.tw. (38103)
93   cochrane database*.jn. (9039)
94   88 or 89 or 90 or 91 or 92 or 93 (112607)
95   15 and 94 (1435)
96   exp brain neoplasms/ (111650)
97   (cancer* or neoplasm* or tumor* or malign*).mp. and brain.tw. (75605)
98   exp Glioma/ (55756)
99   96 or 97 or 98 (164154)
100  15 and 99 (9656)
101  exp pain/ (283152)
102  exp chronic disease/ (210066)
103  101 and 102 (20005)
104  (chronic* adj3 pain*).mp. (32890)
105  103 or 104 (40897)
106  15 and 105 (366)
107  exp sports/ (100542)
108  exp recreation/ (116143)
109  (return* adj3 play*).tw. (803)
110  107 or 108 or 109 (116607)
111  15 and 110 (3782)
112  exp mental disorders/ (880032)
113  15 and 112 (15929)
114  exp disability evaluation/ (35932)
115  exp "Outcome Assessment (Health Care)"/ (605282)
116  disab:.tw. (119042)

117    114 or 115 or 116 (728782)

118    15 and 117 (17459)

119    74 or 85 or 95 or 100 or 106 or 111 or 113 or 118 (68980)

120    limit 119 to (english language and yr=”2001 -Current” and (danish or english or french or norwegian or swedish)) (43016)

121    animals/ not (humans/ and animals/) (3693774)

122    120 not 121 (39793)

123    exp “United States Department of Veterans Affairs”/ or exp Veterans Health/ or exp Hospitals, Veterans/ or exp Veterans Disability Claims/ or exp Veterans/ (15311)

124    veteran.mp. (2331)

125    veterans.mp. (23349)

126    VA.mp. (16805)

127    VA.in. (58986)

128    VAMC.mp. (285)

129    VAMC.in. (2086)

130    exp Military Medicine/ or exp “United States Department of Defense”/ or exp Naval Medicine/ (30814)

131    exp Hospitals, Military/ (3861)

132    exp Military Facilities/ (3901)

133    (army or navy or air force or marines or coast guard).mp. [mp=title, abstract, original title, name of substance word, subject heading word, protocol supplementary concept, rare disease supplementary concept, unique identifier] (15842)

134    military.mp. or exp Military Personnel/ (22947)

135    soldier.mp. (1480)

136    soldiers.mp. (5245)

137    123 or 124 or 125 or 126 or 127 or 128 or 129 or 130 or 131 or 132 or 133 or 134 or 135 or 136 (151164)

138    122 and 137 (1170)

139    traumatic brain injury.mp. or exp Brain Injuries/ (48119)

140    tbi.mp. (10831)

141    139 or 140 (51178)

142    137 and 141 (1468)

143    138 or 142 (1977)

144    from 143 keep 1-1977 (1977)

**************************

The above search strategy was applied to two additional databases on Oct. 3, 2012, with the following yield:

PsycINFO=961

Cochrane Register of Controlled Trials (OVID)=46

# APPENDIX B. STUDY SELECTION FORM

1. Language: Is the full text of the article in English?
   Yes........................................................................................Proceed to #2
   No...........................................................................................Code **X1**. STOP

2. Population: Is the population adult, human participants who are Veterans or members of the military from any country? Studies that do not differentiate between adult and child populations, or between Veteran/military and civilian populations, will be excluded.
   Yes........................................................................................Proceed to #3
   No.................Code **X2**. Add code **B** if retaining for background/discussion. STOP

3. Publication type: Does the article present original study data, or is it a systematic-review or meta-analysis? Narrative or non-systematic reviews, letters, editorials, and commentaries will be excluded.
   Yes........................................................................................Proceed to #4
   No.................Code **X3**. Add code **B** if retaining for background/discussion. STOP

4. Case definition: Does the article stratify/examine mTBI separately from moderate to severe TBI cases? Participants can consist of a mixed group of TBI severity (mild, moderate or severe) only if the results are stratified by severity and the mTBI subjects can be clearly identified. Studies that include mixed groups of TBI severity and do not differentiate between mild, moderate and severe TBI in their analysis will be excluded. Patients must be clearly described as having mTBI, Post-Concussive Syndrome, or concussion; if none of these terms are used, patients must be clearly defined as falling within the definition of mTBI from the VA/DoD Clinical Practice Guideline for Management of Concussion/Mild Traumatic Brain Injury (2009) listed below.
   Yes........................................................................................Proceed to #5
   No.................Code **X4**. Add code **B** if retaining for background/discussion. STOP

5. Systematic review: Is the article a systematic review or meta-analysis of primary studies?
   Yes.......................................................... Code **ISR (systematic review)**. STOP
   No.........................................................................................Proceed to #6

6. Sample size: Is the article a primary study with a sample size of at least 30 mTBI cases?
   Yes........................................................................................Proceed to #7
   No ..............Code **X6**. Add code **B** if retaining for background/discussion. STOP

7. Applicability: Does the study report outcomes addressed in our Key Questions (e.g., health, cognitive, etc. for KQ1; or factors *associated* with outcomes in KQ1; or cost/utilization)?
   Yes........................................................................................Proceed to #8
   No.................Code **X7**. Add code **B** if retaining for background/discussion. STOP

8. Intervention studies: Is the study an intervention study?
   Yes........................................................................................Proceed to #9
   No.........................................................................................Proceed to #10

9.  Intervention outcomes: Does the intervention study report outcomes not influenced by intervention participation (e.g., baseline and/or control group outcome data)?

      Yes.................................................................................Proceed to #10

      No..................Code **X8**. Add code **B** if retaining for background/discussion. STOP

10. VA/DoD mTBI definition: Does the study define mTBI participants as meeting the VA/DoD Clinical Practice Guideline for Management of Concussion/Mild Traumatic Brain Injury (2009) definition of mTBI (listed below) with the exception of including/excluding/not reporting positive imaging results? Studies may use a different mTBI definition, but all criteria with the exception of positive imaging must fall within the VA/DoD definition.

      Yes..................................................................Code **IPS (primary study)**. STOP

      No................Code **X10.** Add code **B** if retaining for background/discussion. STOP

# APPENDIX C. DEFINITION OF MTBI FROM THE VA/DOD CLINICAL PRACTICE GUIDELINE FOR MANAGEMENT OF CONCUSSION/MILD TRAUMATIC BRAIN INJURY (2009)

## 1.1 Definition of Traumatic Brain Injury

A traumatically induced structural injury and/or physiological disruption of brain function as a result of an external force that is indicated by new onset or worsening of at least one of the following clinical signs, immediately following the event:

- Any period of loss of or a decreased level of consciousness (LOC)
- Any loss of memory for events immediately before or after the injury (post-traumatic amnesia[6])
- Any alteration in mental state at the time of the injury (confusion, disorientation, slowed thinking, etc.) (Alteration of consciousness/mental state[5])
- Neurological deficits (weakness, loss of balance, change in vision, praxis, paresis/plegia, sensory loss, aphasia, etc.) that may or may not be transient
- Intracranial lesion

External forces may include any of the following events: the head being struck by an object, the head striking an object, the brain undergoing an acceleration/deceleration movement without direct external trauma to the head, a foreign body penetrating the brain, forces generated from events such as a blast or explosion, or other forces yet to be defined.

The above criteria define the event of a TBI. Not all individuals exposed to an external force will sustain a TBI, but any person who has a history of such an event with immediate manifestation of any of the above signs and symptoms can be said to have had a TBI.

## 1.2 Severity of Brain Injury Stratification

TBI is further categorized as to severity into mild, moderate, or severe based on the length of LOC, AOC, or PTA (see Table A-1). Acute injury severity is determined at the time of the injury.

- The patient is classified as mild/moderate/severe if s/he meets any of the criteria in Table A-1 within a particular severity level. If a patient meets criteria in more than one category of severity, the higher severity level is assigned.
- If it is not clinically possible to determine the brain injury level of severity because of medical complications (e.g., medically induced coma), other severity markers are required to make a determination of the severity of the brain injury.
- Abnormal structural imaging (e.g., Magnetic Resonance Imaging or Computed Tomography Scanning) attributed to the injury will result in the individual being considered clinically to have greater than mild injury.

In addition to traditional imaging studies, other imaging techniques such as functional magnetic resonance imaging, diffusion tensor imaging, positron emission tomography scanning; electrophysiological testing such as electroencephalography; and neuropsychological or other standardized testing of function have been used in the evaluation of persons with TBIs, but are not considered in the currently accepted criteria for measuring severity at the time of the acute injury outlined in Table A -1.

The severity level has prognostic value, but does not necessarily predict the patient's ultimate level of functioning. There is substantial evidence that the epidemiology, pathophysiology, natural history, and prognosis for concussion/mTBI are different than for moderate and severe TBI. For example, moderate and severe TBI are often associated with objective evidence of brain injury on brain scan or neurological examination (e.g., neurological deficits) and objective deficits on neuropsychological testing, whereas these evaluations are frequently not definitive in persons with concussion/mTBI. The natural history and prognosis of moderate and severe TBI are much more directly related to the nature and severity of the injury in moderate and severe TBI, whereas factors unrelated to the injury (such as co-existing mental disorders) have been shown to be the strong predictors of symptom persistence after a concussion/mTBI.

**Table A-1. Classification of TBI Severity**

| Criteria | Mild | Moderate | Severe |
|---|---|---|---|
| Structural imaging | Normal | Normal or abnormal | Normal or abnormal |
| Loss of Consciousness (LOC) | 0–30 min | > 30 min and < 24 hrs | > 24 hrs |
| Alteration of consciousness/ mental state (AOC) | a moment up to 24 hrs | > 24 hours. Severity based on other criteria | |
| Post-traumatic amnesia (PTA) | 0-1 day | > 1 and < 7 days | > 7 days |
| Glasgow Coma Scale (best available score in first 24 hours) | 13-15 | 9-12 | < 9 |

# APPENDIX D. EXCLUDED STUDIES THAT DID NOT MEET MTBI DEFINITION CRITERIA

| Author, Year | Definition | Patients with Abnormal Imaging | Citation | How Assessed |
|---|---|---|---|---|
| Adams, Larson, Corrigan, et al., 2012[1] | Length of LOC classified as < 1 minute, 1-20 minutes, or > 20 minutes. Used the Health Related Behaviors Among Active Duty Military Personnel Survey response categories: "The HRB Survey symptom response groups permit recoding LOC as up to 20 minutes and greater than 20 minutes. This provides insufficient information to code LOC using the American Congress of Rehabilitation Medicine's definition of mild TBI." | NR | Kay, Harrington, Adams, et al., 1993 | Self-report survey |
| Arbisi, Polusny, Erbes, et al., 2011[2] | Adapted from the Defense and Veterans Brain Injury Center screening tool: yes to last item "dazed, confused, see stars, get knocked out or lose consciousness" classified as mTBI. No participants reported "receiving treatment while in Iraq for a TBI or were removed from assigned duties as a result of exposure to blast or other form of head trauma." | NR | Schwab et al., 2007 | Self-report mailed questionnaire |
| Armistead-Jehle, 2010[3] | "Screened positive on the VHA TBI screens" for "possible mTBI." "All patients suffered at most a mild TBI..., as none reported loss of consciousness of more than 30 minutes or posttraumatic amnesia of 24 hours or more." | NR | US Department of Veterans Affairs, 2007 | Self-report |
| Bazarian, Donnelly, Peterson, et al., 2012[4] | "Mild TBI diagnosis was determined by in-person interview using a 22-item questionnaire developed to establish the nature, probability, and severity of deployment-related TBI among OEF/OIF veterans. The interview followed previously published TBI diagnostic criteria, which include confirmation of a possible TBI event, confirmation of alteration of consciousness, and confirmation of postconcussion symptoms. On the basis of the standardized clinical interview, interviewers rated the likelihood of mild TBI according to a 6-point scale: "not at all likely," "very unlikely," "somewhat unlikely," "somewhat likely," "very likely," and "almost certainly." These likelihood categories were used in all analyses. However, for descriptive purposes, subjects were defined as having mild TBI if interviewers rated them "very likely" or "almost certainly."" | NR | Lew, Poole, & Vanderploeg, 2007 | Clinical interview |

| Author, Year | Definition | Patients with Abnormal Imaging | Citation | How Assessed |
|---|---|---|---|---|
| Booth-Kewley, Highfill-McRoy, Larson, et al., 2012[5] | "Mild TBI symptoms were assessed using a set of questions that asked participants whether they had received an injury to the head during their most recent deployment that involved 'being dazed, confused, or 'seeing stars'' or 'not remembering the injury, or losing consciousness (knocked out).' A participant was classified as having a positive TBI screen if any of the three questions elicited a positive response." | NR | Centers for Disease Control and Prevention & World Health Organization definitions adapted by the Defense and Veterans Brain Injury Center working group for military use | Self-report survey |
| Brenner, Terrio, Homaifar, et al., 2010[6] | Warrior Administered Retrospective Casualty Assessment Tool (WARCAT) and Brief Trauma Brain Injury Screen. "All 45 participants whose test scores were included in analyses had a history of blast exposure with alteration of or loss of consciousness (LOC)." "The nature of the most serious mTBIs reported were: $n = 30$, altered consciousness only; $n = 12$, up to 1-min LOC; and $n = 3$, one to 20-min LOC." | NR | Soldier Readiness Process, 2007; Schwab et al., 2007 | Chart review, self-report survey, and clinical interview |
| Brenner, Ivins, Schwab, Warden, Nelson, Jaffee, & Terrio, 2010[7] | As described in Terrio et al., 2009: Warrior Administered Retrospective Casualty Assessment Tool (WARCAT) and Brief Trauma Brain Injury Screen | NR | Soldier Readiness Process, 2007; Schwab et al., 2007 | Chart review, self-report survey, and clinical interview |
| Cameron, Marshall, Sturdivant, & Lincoln, 2011[8] | "Incident cases of mTBI were operationally defined according to the administrative case definition proposed by the Centers for Disease Control and Prevention (CDC) for research purposes... and include ICD-9-CM codes for skull fracture (800.00, 800.5, 801.0, 801.5, 803.0, 803.5, 804.0, and 804.5), concussion (850.0, 850.1, 850.5, and 850.9), intracranial injury of unspecified nature (854.0), and head injury unspecified (959.01). In addition to the four digit codes listed, all subordinate five-digit codes were also included." | NR | Centers for Disease Control and Prevention, 2003 | Chart review |
| Carlson, Kehle, Meis, et al., 2011[9] | "Included studies must have assessed participants for a "probable" TBI (identified using self-report screening instruments) or diagnosed TBI history." | NR | NR | NA |
| Clement & Kennedy, 2003[10] | LOC<60 minutes with no neurological findings | Excluded | NR | Chart review |

| Author, Year | Definition | Patients with Abnormal Imaging | Citation | How Assessed |
|---|---|---|---|---|
| Dougherty, MacGregor, Han, et al., 2011[11] | International Classification of Diseases, 9th Revision (ICD-9) codes 800.0-801.9, 803.0-804.9, 850.0-854.1. "The Abbreviated Injury Scale (AIS) was used to describe the severity of brain injury... Due to a small number of TBI observations with scores of 4 (severe injury) and 5 (critical injury) in the present study, TBI severity was classified as follows: 0 = No TBI, 1 = minor, 2 = moderate and 3-5 = serious to critical. Service members with AIS scores of 6 were not eligible for inclusion in the study." | NR | Gennarelli & Wodzin, 2005 | Chart review |
| Drake, Gray, Yoder, et al., 2000[12] | "Subjects were consecutive MTBI patients... meeting specific inclusion criteria... a documented TBI classified by accepted criteria as a mild TBI." No specific mTBI definition noted. | NR | NR | Self-report and chart review |
| Eskridge, 2011[13] | "Clinical diagnosis codes from the International Classification of Diseases, 9th Revision (ICD-9) were assigned to each injury... In addition to the assigning of diagnosis codes, severity of each injury is accessed with two different standardized measures of injury severity; the Abbreviated Injury Scale (AIS) and the Injury Severity Scale (ISS)... The ISS for each blast episode was documented and categorized into one of four severity levels; mild (ISS 1-3), moderate (ISS 4-8), serious (ISS 9-15) and severe (ISS 16 and higher)." | NR | NR | Chart review |
| Fear, Jones, Groom, et al., 2009[14] | "Criteria for identification include confusion or disorientation, loss of consciousness lasting less than 30 min or post-traumatic amnesia lasting less than 24 h." However, description of population studied only states, "we have examined the prevalence of symptoms thought to be a consequence of mTBI," with unclear description of how mTBI was determined. | NR | Holm, et al., 2005 | Chart review |
| Ferrier-Auerbach, Erbes, Polusny, et al., 2009[15] | "Three items adapted from the Defense and Veterans Brain Injury Center (DVBIC) Blast Exposure Screening Questionnaire... (1) Were you ever so close to a blast that you could feel the blast wave (such as heat or pressure) or afterward had trouble hearing or problems with attention or memory?... (2) Did you have any injuries from a blast, vehicle crash, bullet/shrapnel or fall?... (3) Did any injury cause you to be dazed/confused, 'see stars,' get knocked out, or lose consciousness?" | NR | Schwab et al., 2007 | Self-report survey |

| Author, Year | Definition | Patients with Abnormal Imaging | Citation | How Assessed |
|---|---|---|---|---|
| French, Lange, Iverson, Ivins, et al., 2012[16] | LOC < 15 mins; PTA < 24 hours; absence of intracranial abnormality on computed tomography or magnetic resonance imaging scan | Excluded | Used VA/DoD criteria, but data limited to LOC < 15 minute categories. | Chart review |
| Gottshall, Gray, Drake, et al., 2007[17] | Definition: GCS 13-15. One patient identified as having an open head injury. LOC categorized as 31-60 (1 patient), and > 60 minutes (one patient), and up to 20 minutes (all remaining patients). | NR | American Academy of Neurology, 1997 | Clinical presentation (to ED or Battalion Aid Station) |
| Helfer, Jordan, Lee, et al., 2011[18] | ICD-9CM codes 850.0, 850.11, 850.12, 850.2, 850.3, 850.4, 850.5, 850.9, 959.01, V15.52 | NR | US Dept of Health and Human Services, 2008 | Chart review |
| Heltemes, Dougherty, MacGregor, & Galarneau, 2011[19] | International Classification of Diseases, 9th Revision, Clinical Modification (ICD-9-CM) codes 800.0-801.9, 803.0-804.9, 850.0-854.1. | NR | Centers for Disease Control and Prevention, 2003 | Chart review |
| Hoffer, Balaban, Gottshall, et al., 2010[20] | "Definitive diagnosis of mild traumatic brain as defined by the 2007 Joint Service Surgeon General's Definition" | NR | Assistant Secretary of Defense: Memorandum on Traumatic Brain Injury: Definition and Reporting. Available at http://www.pdhealth.mil/TBI.asp | In theater clinical evaluation |
| Hoffer, Donaldson, Gottshall, et al., 2009[21] | No specific mTBI definition listed. | NR | NR | Clinical interview |
| Hoge, McGurk, Thomas, et al., 2008[22] | Positive response to three questions: LOC, being dazed and confused, seeing stars or not remembering the injury. However, "four Soldiers reported LOC lasting longer than 30 minutes. Although technically they were considered to have a moderate TBI they were not excluded because the number was low and it was not possible to verify the self-report data on any of the subjects". | NR | DVBIC, 2006; CDC, 2003 | Self-report |
| Ivins, Schwab, Baker, & Warden, 2003[23] | "Head injury for which any LOC or any alteration of mental state without LOC was reported." Reports rates of concussion grades separately, though the categories are divided by LOC < 20 minutes and LOC between 20-59 minutes. | NR | Kay et al., 1993 | Chart review |
| Ivins, Schwab, Baker, & Warden, 2006[24] | ICD-9CM codes 800.00-801.99, 803.00-804.99, and 850.0-854.19 and AIS severity codes of minor or moderate. | NR | Kay et al., 1993; Thurman & Guerrero, 1999 | Chart review |

| Author, Year | Definition | Patients with Abnormal Imaging | Citation | How Assessed |
|---|---|---|---|---|
| Ivins, Kane, & Schwab, 2009[25] | Brief Traumatic Brain Injury Screen (BTBIS); LOC criteria < 20 mins. Additional computerized survey administered; however, it appears that only those with LOC < 20 minutes were included in the further assessment. Brief Traumatic Brain Injury Screen (BTBIS); Patients who screened positive for TBI and had LOC< = 20 minutes and/or possible PTA< = 24 hours were identified as having MTBI with LOC or possible PTA | NR | Kay et al., 1993; Thurman & Guerrero, 1999 | Chart review |
| Ivins, 2010[26] | Mapped ICD-9 CM diagnoses to the Abbreviated Injury Scale (AIS): ICD-9CM codes 800.00-801.99, 803.00-804.99, and 850.0-854.19 and AIS severity codes of minor or moderate. Combines mild and moderate into one category. | NR | Kay et al., 1993; Thurman & Guerrero, 1999 | Chart review |
| Lange, Pancholi, Bhagwat, et al., 2012[27] | "PTA < 24 hours and LOC < 15 minutes." "It was our preference to use a LOC criterion of < 30 minutes, consistent with commonly used diagnostic criteria... However, the available information regarding LOC was limited to categorical data that did not allow us to differentiate between LOC greater or lower than 30 min." | Included | Carroll et al., 2004; Management of Concussion/mTBI Working Group, 2009; ACRM, 1993 | Chart review |
| Lange, Pancholi, Brickell, et al., 2012[28] | LOC < 15 mins; PTA < 24 hours | Included | Used VA/DoD criteria, but data limited to LOC < 15 minute categories. | Chart review and clinical interview |
| Lange, Brickell, French, et al., 2012[29] | Uncomplicated: PTA<24 hours, LOC < 15 mins, negative imaging; complicated: positive imaging. "It was our preference to use an LOC criterion of 30 min to classify MTBI consistent with commonly used military and civilian diagnostic criteria. However, the available information regarding LOC was limited to categorical data that did not allow us to differentiate between LOC greater or less than 30 min (i.e., available data = LOC < 15 min and LOC 16–60 min)." | Excluded | Used VA/DoD criteria, but data limited to LOC < 15 minute categories. | Routine comprehensive clinical evaluation |
| Lew, Garvert, Pogoda, et al., 2009[30] | Mild TBI was defined as an initial GCS score of 13 to 15, PTA duration of <1 day, or LOC duration of <1 hour | NR | NR | Chart review and clinical evaluation |

| Author, Year | Definition | Patients with Abnormal Imaging | Citation | How Assessed |
|---|---|---|---|---|
| Luis, Venderploeg, & Curtiss, 2003[31] | "During the interview, participants were asked, among many others, the following three questions: 1) since your discharge from active duty, have you been injured in a MVA? 2) Since your discharge from active duty have you injured your head (HI)? and (3) Did you lose consciousness as a result of the head injury?"<br>Analysis by LOC group but time of LOC not specified. | NR | NR | Self-report |
| MacGregor, 2007[32] | "An ICD-9 code in the following ranges was defined as a TBI (n = 124): 800.0-801.9 (fractures of the vault or base of the skull); 803.0-804.9 (other and unqualified and multiple fractures of the skull); and 850.0-854.1 (intracranial injury, including concussion, contusion, laceration, and hemorrhage)... Severity of TBI was indicated with the Abbreviated Injury Scale (AIS). The AIS ranges from 1 (relatively minor) to 6 (currently untreatable), and is determined separately for each different body region. Severity of TBI was determined by maximum AIS score for the head region – head AIS 1-2 indicated mild TBI, head AIS 3-5 indicated moderate-severe TBI. A majority of TBI identified via CHAMPS did not have a head AIS score present; in this case the TBI was assumed to be of mild severity due to a closed head injury." | NR | ICD-9-CM, 2005 | Chart review |
| MacGregor, Dougherty, & Galarneau, 2011[33] | International Classification of Diseases, 9th Revision (ICD-9) codes 800.0-801.9, 803.0-804.9, 850.0-854.1. "The AIS was used to describe the severity of these injuries and the injuries were scored according to the following scale: 0, no injury; 1 minor; 2, moderate; 3, serious; 4, severe; 5, critical; 6, fatal injury. As per previous literature, each participant was categorized by the severity of their highest (or maximum) AIS Head score as mild (AIS score = 1-2), moderate (AIS score = 3), or severe (AIS score = 4-6). | NR | Ommaya, Ommaya, Dannenberg, et al., 1996 | Chart review |
| MacGregor, Dougherty, Morrison, et al., 2011[34] | "A concussion was defined by the ICD-9-CM code of 850.0-850.9. Severity of concussion was defined using the AIS." | NR | NR | Chart review |
| MacGregor, Shaffer, Dougherty, et al. 2010[35] | ICD-9 codes 800-801.9, 803-804.9, and 850-854.1; Abbreviated Injury Scale (AIS) score 1-2 = "mild," 3-5 = "moderate to severe" | NR | Ommaya et al., 1996 | Chart review |

| Author, Year | Definition | Patients with Abnormal Imaging | Citation | How Assessed |
|---|---|---|---|---|
| McGuire, Marsh, Sowin, & Robinson, 2012[36] | "LOC less than 30 min or amnesia less than 60 min" | NR | Annegers et al., 1998 | NR |
| Mora, Ritenour, Wade, et al., 2009[37] | "Consciousness status to determine mTBI was queried using both codes from ICD and Abbreviated Injury Scale for indications of trauma to the head, concussive injuries, and indications of consciousness at the time of injury. A loss of consciousness served as the definition for mTBI. | NR | NR | Chart review |
| Morgan, Lockwood, Steinke, et al., 2012[38] | No clear mTBI definition. | NR | NR | Self-report screening and clinical interview |
| Nelson, Weiser, Giford, et al., 2011[39] | "The Brief Traumatic Brain Injury Screen was used to identify cases (probable mTBI) and controls (no mTBI). Individuals were placed in the "probable mTBI" group if they endorsed an injury (reported at least one injury on the BTBIS) and indicated that they had lost consciousness for a defined period of time (ranging from less than 1 minute to longer than 20 minutes) following the injury. Those who did not report an injury or a loss of consciousness (LOC) for any amount of time following an injury acted as the control group." | NR | Defense and Veterans Brain Injury Center (DVBIC) | Chart review |
| Olson-Madden, Forster, Huggins, & Schneider, 2012[40] | "Injury severity data were coded as either mild (alteration in consciousness or loss of consciousness $</=$ 30 minutes) or moderate/severe (loss of consciousness > 30 minutes)." | NR | Kay et al., 1993 | Clinical interview |
| Ommaya, Ommaya, Dannenberg, et al., 1996[41] | "Head-injury-related discharge diagnosis (800.00-801.99, 803.00-804.99, and 850.0-854.19)." Injury Severity Scale and Abbreviated Injury Scale were calculated. | NR | NR | Chart review |
| Ommaya, Salazar, Dannenberg, et al., 1996[42] | "Records with a head-injury hospital-related discharge diagnosis (800.00-801.99, 803.00-804.99, and 850.0-854.19) were identified as described in a previous study." "Maximum Abbreviated Injury Score (AIS) head and Injury Severity Score (ISS) were computed using the ICD-9 map. Mild TBI was defined as maximum AIS head equal to 1 or 2" | NR | NR | Clinical records |
| Pietrzak, Johnson, Goldstein, Malley, Southwick 2009[43] | "Positive mTBI screen" based on endorsement of all 4 items on the DVBIC questionnaire | NR | GAO, 2008 & DVBIC, 2006 | Self-report survey |

| Author, Year | Definition | Patients with Abnormal Imaging | Citation | How Assessed |
|---|---|---|---|---|
| Plassman, Havlik, Steffens, et al., 2000[44] | "1) mild injury = loss of consciousness or posttraumatic amnesia for less than 30 minutes, with no skull fracture; 2) moderate injury = loss of consciousness or post-traumatic amnesia for more than 30 minutes but less than 24 hours, and/or a skull fracture; and 3) severe injury = loss of consciousness or post-traumatic amnesia for more than 24 hours." | NR | Frankowski, Annengers, & Whitman, 1985 | Chart review |
| Polusny, Kehle, Nelson, Erbes, Arbisi, Thuras, 2011[45] | Injury with altered mental status or LOC (items 1-3 on DVBIC screen) | NR | Schwab et al., 2007 | Self-report in theater, 1 month prior to return home |
| Roebuck-Spencer, Vincent, Twille, et al., 2012[46] | "Although data on recency and severity of injury were not available in this dataset, TBIs reported in this study are presumed to be mild in nature given that Service Members were still on active duty. Mild TBI was defined as such when individuals reported an injury event accompanied by an alteration of consciousness. This included endorsement of at least one of the following: feeling dazed or confused, experiencing loss of consciousness (LOC), or experiencing loss of memory for the injury or posttraumatic amnesia (PTA) for the event." | NR | NR | Self-report screening tool |
| Romesser, Shen, Reblin, Kircher, Allen, Roberts, & Marchand, 2011[47] | "History of military-related concussion during a VHA TBI secondary evaluation." Excluded if "self-report suggested a history of a moderate or severe TBI (i.e., if they endorsed loss of consciousness more than 30 minutes)." | NR | NR | Clinical interview |
| Rona, Jones, Fear, et al., 2012[48] | "Possible mTBI was assessed using a modified version of the BTBIS... A second item asked about possible symptoms associated with the injury. These were losing consciousness; being dazed or confused; not remembering the injury; concussion (e.g., headache, dizziness); head injury, and none of these. Participants were asked to tick all that applied. Self-report of the duration of any loss of consciousness was also obtained, we eliminated one participant from the analysis who reported prolonged loss of consciousness... Participants who endorsed at least one of these symptoms were classified as having mTBI." | NR | Iverson, Langlois, McCrea, & Kelly, 2009 | Self-report question-naire |

| Author, Year | Definition | Patients with Abnormal Imaging | Citation | How Assessed |
|---|---|---|---|---|
| Rona, Jones, Fear, et al., 2012[49] | "Possible mTBI was assessed using a modified version of the BTBIS, which included an item exploring possible causes of injury (blast, shrapnel fragments, bullet, fall, and vehicle accident and other). Participants could state that they had not suffered an injury during deployment. A second item asked about possible symptoms associated with the injury. These were losing consciousness; being dazed or confused; not remembering the injury; concussion (e.g., headache, dizziness); head injury; and none of these. Participants were asked to tick all that applied. Self-report of the duration of any loss of consciousness was also obtained, we eliminated 1 participant from the analysis who reported prolonged loss of consciousness (which would be classified traumatic brain injury, not mTBI). Participants who endorsed at least one of these symptoms were classified as having mTBI." | NR | Iverson, Langlois, McCrea, & Kelly, 2009 | Self-report question-naire |
| Schneiderman, Braver & Kang, 2008[50] | Three-item Brief Traumatic Brain Injury Screen | NR | Defense and Veterans Brain Injury Center | Self-report survey |
| Skopp, Trofimovich, Grimes, et al., 2012[51] | mild TBI (subset of all TBI codes): 310.2, 800.00-800.02, 800.06, 800.09, 800.50, 800.52, 801.00, 801.01,801.02, 801.06, 801.09, 801.50, 801.51, 801.52, 803.00-803.02, 803.06, 803.09, 803.50, 803.51, 803.52, 804.00, 804.01, 804.02, 804.06, 804.09, 804.50, 804.51, 804.52, 850.0, 805.1, 850.11, 850.9, 959.01, V15.52, V15.5_7, V15.5_C, V15.52_2, V15.52_2,V15.52_7, V15.52_C | NR | DoD standard TBI surveillance case definition to ascertain TBI status and severity | Chart review |

| Author, Year | Definition | Patients with Abnormal Imaging | Citation | How Assessed |
|---|---|---|---|---|
| Theeler, Flynn, & Erickson, 2010[52] | "2-question screen followed by a 10-question screen… The first question asks if, while deployed, the soldier was exposed to or near a blast, improvised explosive device (IED) explosion, car bomb, suicide explosion, or exposed to any other combat event or resulted in a blow or jolt to the head. The second question asks if the soldier was involved in a motor vehicle accident, a fall, a sports accident, or any other event that caused a blow to the head or resulted in a neck whiplash. If the soldier answers yes to either question 1 or 2, 10 more questions asking about loss of consciousness, dazed sensation after the event, and neurologic or behavioral sequelae following the event are administered. This questionnaire is scored in a standardized manner from 0 to 39. The case definition for concussion constituted a score of 5 or greater on the 2-plus-10 questionnaire." | NR | NR | Self-report survey |
| Theeler, Flynn, & Erickson, 2012[53] | No specific criteria: 2-question followed by a 10-question screen if the soldier answers yes to either of the first 2 questions. This questionnaire is scored in a standardized manner from 0 to 39; the score from the 2-plus-10 questionnaire will herein be called the TBI Score | NR | Theeler, Flynn, & Erickson, 2010 | Self-report survey |
| Vanderploeg, Belanger, & Curtiss, 2009[54] | "Have you injured your head?... Did you lose consciousness as a result of the head injury?" "those individuals who required hospitalization after their head injury (n = 40) were excluded." "head injury with altered consciousness" were classified as mild TBI. | NR | NR | Clinical interview |
| Vanderploeg, Curtiss & Belanger, 2005[55] | "During the interview, participants were asked, among many others, the following three questions: 1) Since your discharge from active duty, have you been injured in a MVA? 2) Since your discharge from active duty have you injured your head (HI)? and 3) Did you lose consciousness as a result of the head injury?" | NR | NR | Self-report |
| Vanderploeg, Curtiss, Duchnick, Luis, 2003[56] | Positive responses to following questions: "Since discharge from active duty, have you been injured in a MVA?"; "Since discharge from active duty, have you injured your head (from any cause)?"; and "Did you lose consciousness as a result of the head injury?" | NR | NR | Self-report survey |

| Author, Year | Definition | Patients with Abnormal Imaging | Citation | How Assessed |
|---|---|---|---|---|
| Vasterling, Brailey, Proctor, et al., 2012[57] | "Congruent with reports showing stronger associations between clinical outcomes and TBI following loss of consciousness v. altered consciousness, only those pre- to post-deployment interval injuries resulting in loss of consciousness were queried." | NR | NR | Self-report survey |
| Wilk, Herrell, Wynn, Riviere, & Hoge, 2012[58] | "Injury resulted in being dazed, confused, or seeing stars, not remembering the injury, or losing consciousness (knocked out)." | NR | DoD/VA Brain Injury Center Brief Traumatic Brain Injury Screen | Self-report survey |
| Wilk, Thomas, McGurk, et al., 2010[59] | "Injury resulted in being dazed, confused, or seeing stars, not remembering the injury, or losing consciousness (knocked out)." | NR | DoD/VA Brain Injury Center Brief Traumatic Brain Injury Screen | Self-report survey |
| Yurkiewicz, Lappan, Neely, et al., 2012[60] | "Defense and Veterans Brain Injury Center (DVBIC) assesses TBI severity after a blast event or motor vehicle accident, answers questions about evacuation and in-theater clinical care and medication, and provides recommendations on headache management and vision, hearing, vestibular, and neurologic issues. Successes of the program include a stratified headache protocol for primary care providers and an early management protocol for mild TBI and posttraumatic headache stratified headache protocol." "We reviewed consults sent to the neurology group from October 2006 to December 2010 and consults sent to the TBI group from March 2008 to December 2010. Microsoft Excel spreadsheets were constructed to organize and analyze data regarding number of consultations, response times, location of origin, branch of service, clinical images transmitted, anatomic location of complaint, type of injury, workup recommended, and treatment and evacuation recommendations." | NR | DVBIC Brief Traumatic Brain Injury Screen | Chart review |

*Note.* None of the studies reported information on assessor blinding of study hypotheses when assessing mTBI.

**Bibliography of studies excluded for not meeting mTBI definition criteria**

1.   Adams RS, Larson MJ, Corrigan JD, Horgan CM, Williams TV. Frequent binge drinking after combat-acquired traumatic brain injury among active duty military personnel with a past year combat deployment. *J Head Trauma Rehabil.* Sep 2012;27(5):349-360.

2.   Arbisi PA, Polusny MA, Erbes CR, Thuras P, Reddy MK. The Minnesota Multiphasic Personality Inventory-2 Restructured Form in National Guard soldiers screening positive for posttraumatic stress disorder and mild traumatic brain injury. *Psychol Assess.* Mar 2011;23(1):203-214.

3.   Armistead-Jehle P. Symptom validity test performance in U.S. veterans referred for evaluation of mild TBI. *Appl Neuropsychol.* Jan 2010;17(1):52-59.

4.   Bazarian JJ, Zhu T, Blyth B, Borrino A, Zhong J. Subject-specific changes in brain white matter on diffusion tensor imaging after sports-related concussion. *Magn Reson Imaging.* Feb 2012;30(2):171-180.

5.   Booth-Kewley S, Highfill-McRoy RM, Larson GE, Garland CF, Gaskin TA. Anxiety and depression in marines sent to war in iraq and afghanistan. *J Nerv Ment Dis.* Sep 2012;200(9):749-757.

6.   Brenner LA, Terrio H, Homaifar BY, et al. Neuropsychological test performance in soldiers with blast-related mild TBI. *Neuropsychology.* Mar 2010;24(2):160-167.

7.   Brenner LA, Ivins BJ, Schwab K, et al. Traumatic brain injury, posttraumatic stress disorder, and postconcussive symptom reporting among troops returning from iraq. *J Head Trauma Rehabil.* Sep-Oct 2010;25(5):307-312.

8.   Cameron KL, Marshall SW, Sturdivant RX, Lincoln AE. Trends in the incidence of physician-diagnosed mild traumatic brain injury among active duty U.S. military personnel between 1997 and 2007. *J Neurotrauma.* May 2012;29(7):1313-1321.

9.   Carlson KF, Kehle SM, Meis LA, et al. Prevalence, assessment, and treatment of mild traumatic brain injury and posttraumatic stress disorder: a systematic review of the evidence. *J Head Trauma Rehabil.* Mar-Apr 2011;26(2):103-115.

10.  Clement PF, Kennedy JE. Wechsler Adult Intelligence Scale-third edition characteristics of a military traumatic brain injury sample. *Mil Med.* Dec 2003;168(12):1025-1028.

11.  Dougherty AL, MacGregor AJ, Han PP, Heltemes KJ, Galarneau MR. Visual dysfunction following blast-related traumatic brain injury from the battlefield. *Brain Inj.* 2011;25(1):8-13.

12.  Drake AI, Gray N, Yoder S, Pramuka M, Llewellyn M. Factors predicting return to work following mild traumatic brain injury: A discriminant analysis. *The Journal of Head Trauma Rehabilitation.* Oct 2000;15(5):1103-1112.

13.  Eskridge SL. Combat-related blast injuries: Injury types and outcomes. *Dissertation Abstracts International: Section B: The Sciences and Engineering.* 2012;72(7-B):3929.

14. Fear N, Jones E, Groom M, et al. Symptoms of post-concussional syndrome are nonspecifically related to mild traumatic brain injury in UK Armed Forces personnel on return from deployment in Iraq: An analysis of self-reported data. *Psychological Medicine.* Aug 2009;39(8):1379-1387.

15. Ferrier-Auerbach AG, Erbes CR, Polusny MA, Rath CM, Sponheim SR. Predictors of emotional distress reported by soldiers in the combat zone. *J Psychiatr Res.* May 2010;44(7):470-476.

16. French LM, Lange RT, Iverson GL, Ivins B, Marshall K, Schwab K. Influence of bodily injuries on symptom reporting following uncomplicated mild traumatic brain injury in US military service members. *J Head Trauma Rehabil.* Jan-Feb 2012;27(1):63-74.

17. Gottshall KR, Gray NL, Drake AI, Tejidor R, Hoffer ME, McDonald EC. To investigate the influence of acute vestibular impairment following mild traumatic brain injury on subsequent ability to remain on activity duty 12 months later. *Mil Med.* Aug 2007;172(8):852-857.

18. Helfer TM, Jordan NN, Lee RB, Pietrusiak P, Cave K, Schairer K. Noise-induced hearing injury and comorbidities among postdeployment U.S. Army soldiers: April 2003-June 2009. *Am J Audiol.* Jun 2011;20(1):33-41.

19. Heltemes KJ, Dougherty AL, MacGregor AJ, Galarneau MR. Alcohol abuse disorders among U.S. service members with mild traumatic brain injury. *Mil Med.* Feb 2011;176(2):147-150.

20. Hoffer ME, Balaban C, Gottshall K, Balough BJ, Maddox MR, Penta JR. Blast exposure: vestibular consequences and associated characteristics. *Otol Neurotol.* Feb 2010;31(2):232-236.

21. Hoffer ME, Donaldson C, Gottshall KR, Balaban C, Balough BJ. Blunt and blast head trauma: different entities. *Int Tinnitus J.* 2009;15(2):115-118.

22. Hoge CW, McGurk D, Thomas JL, Cox AL, Engel CC, Castro CA. Mild traumatic brain injury in U.S. Soldiers returning from Iraq. *N Engl J Med.* Jan 31 2008;358(5):453-463.

23. Ivins BJ, Schwab KA, Warden D, et al. Traumatic brain injury in U.S. Army paratroopers: prevalence and character. *J Trauma.* Oct 2003;55(4):617-621.

24. Ivins BJ, Schwab KA, Baker G, Warden DL. Hospital admissions associated with traumatic brain injury in the US Army during peacetime: 1990s trends. *Neuroepidemiology.* 2006;27(3):154-163.

25. Ivins BJ, Kane R, Schwab KA. Performance on the Automated Neuropsychological Assessment Metrics in a nonclinical sample of soldiers screened for mild TBI after returning from Iraq and Afghanistan: a descriptive analysis. *J Head Trauma Rehabil.* Jan-Feb 2009;24(1):24-31.

26. Ivins BJ. Hospitalization associated with traumatic brain injury in the active duty US Army: 2000-2006. *NeuroRehabilitation.* 2010;26(3):199-212.

27. Lange RT, Pancholi S, Bhagwat A, Anderson-Barnes V, French LM. Influence of poor effort on neuropsychological test performance in U.S. military personnel following mild traumatic brain injury. *J Clin Exp Neuropsychol.* 2012;34(5):453-466.

28. Lange RT, Pancholi S, Brickell TA, et al. Neuropsychological Outcome from Blast versus Non-blast: Mild Traumatic Brain Injury in U.S. Military Service Members. *J Int Neuropsychol Soc.* May 2012;18(3):595-605.

29. Lange RT, Brickell TA, French LM, et al. Neuropsychological Outcome from Uncomplicated Mild, Complicated Mild, and Moderate Traumatic Brain Injury in US Military Personnel. *Arch Clin Neuropsychol.* 2012;27(5):480-494.

30. Lew HL, Garvert DW, Pogoda TK, et al. Auditory and visual impairments in patients with blast-related traumatic brain injury: Effect of dual sensory impairment on Functional Independence Measure. *J Rehabil Res Dev.* 2009;46(6):819-826.

31. Luis CA, Vanderploeg RD, Curtiss G. Predictors of postconcussion symptom complex in community dwelling male veterans. *J Int Neuropsychol Soc.* Nov 2003;9(7):1001-1015.

32. Macgregor AJ. Physical injury and psychological outcomes among United States combat veterans. *Dissertation Abstracts International: Section B: The Sciences and Engineering.* 2007;68(6-B):3665.

33. MacGregor AJ, Dougherty AL, Galarneau MR. Injury-specific correlates of combat-related traumatic brain injury in Operation Iraqi Freedom. *The Journal of Head Trauma Rehabilitation.* Jul-Aug 2011;26(4):312-318.

34. MacGregor AJ, Dougherty AL, Morrison RH, Quinn KH, Galarneau MR. Repeated concussion among U.S. military personnel during Operation Iraqi Freedom. *J Rehabil Res Dev.* 2011;48(10):1269-1278.

35. MacGregor AJ, Shaffer RA, Dougherty AL, et al. Prevalence and psychological correlates of traumatic brain injury in operation iraqi freedom. *J Head Trauma Rehabil.* Jan-Feb 2010;25(1):1-8.

36. McGuire SA, Marsh RW, Sowin TW, Robinson AY. Aeromedical decision making and seizure risk after traumatic brain injury: longitudinal outcome. *Aviat Space Environ Med.* Feb 2012;83(2):140-143.

37. Mora AG, Ritenour AE, Wade CE, Holcomb JB, Blackbourne LH, Gaylord KM. Posttraumatic stress disorder in combat casualties with burns sustaining primary blast and concussive injuries. *J Trauma.* Apr 2009;66(4 Suppl):S178-185.

38. Morgan M, Lockwood A, Steinke D, Schleenbaker R, Botts S. Pharmacotherapy regimens among patients with posttraumatic stress disorder and mild traumatic brain injury. *Psychiatric Services.* Feb 2012;63(2):182-185.

39. Nelson C, St, Weiser M, Gifford S, Gallimore J, Morningstar A. Knowledge gained from the Traumatic Brain Injury Screen-Implications for treating Canadian military personnel. *Mil Med.* Feb 2011;176(2):156-160.

40. Olson-Madden JH, Forster JE, Huggins J, Schneider A. Psychiatric diagnoses, mental health utilization, high-risk behaviors, and self-directed violence among veterans with comorbid history of traumatic brain injury and substance use disorders. *J Head Trauma Rehabil.* Sep 2012;27(5):370-378.

41. Ommaya AK, Ommaya AK, Dannenberg AL, Salazar AM. Causation, incidence, and costs of traumatic brain injury in the U.S. military medical system. *J Trauma.* Feb 1996;40(2):211-217.

42. Ommaya AK, Salazar AM, Dannenberg AL, Chervinsky AB, Schwab K. Outcome after traumatic brain injury in the U.S. military medical system. *J Trauma.* Dec 1996;41(6):972-975.

43. Pietrzak RH, Johnson DC, Goldstein MB, Malley JC, Southwick SM. Posttraumatic stress disorder mediates the relationship between mild traumatic brain injury and health and psychosocial functioning in veterans of Operations Enduring Freedom and Iraqi Freedom. *J Nerv Ment Dis.* Oct 2009;197(10):748-753.

44. Plassman BL, Havlik RJ, Steffens DC, et al. Documented head injury in early adulthood and risk of Alzheimer's disease and other dementias. *Neurology.* Oct 24 2000;55(8):1158-1166.

45. Polusny MA, Kehle SM, Nelson NW, Erbes CR, Arbisi PA, Thuras P. Longitudinal effects of mild traumatic brain injury and posttraumatic stress disorder comorbidity on postdeployment outcomes in national guard soldiers deployed to Iraq. *Arch Gen Psychiatry.* Jan 2011;68(1):79-89.

46. Roebuck-Spencer TM, Vincent AS, Twillie DA, et al. Cognitive change associated with self-reported mild traumatic brain injury sustained during the OEF/OIF conflicts. *The Clinical Neuropsychologist.* Apr 2012;26(3):473-489.

47. Romesser J, Shen S, Reblin M, et al. A preliminary study of the effect of a diagnosis of concussion on PTSD symptoms and other psychiatric variables at the time of treatment seeking among veterans. *Mil Med.* Mar 2011;176(3):246-252.

48. Rona RJ, Jones M, Fear NT, et al. Mild traumatic brain injury in UK military personnel returning from Afghanistan and Iraq: cohort and cross-sectional analyses. *J Head Trauma Rehabil.* Jan-Feb 2012;27(1):33-44.

49. Rona RJ, Jones M, Fear NT, Sundin J, Hull L, Wessely S. Frequency of mild traumatic brain injury in Iraq and Afghanistan: are we measuring incidence or prevalence? *J Head Trauma Rehabil.* Jan-Feb 2012;27(1):75-82.

50. Schneiderman AI, Braver ER, Kang HK. Understanding sequelae of injury mechanisms and mild traumatic brain injury incurred during the conflicts in Iraq and Afghanistan: persistent postconcussive symptoms and posttraumatic stress disorder. *Am J Epidemiol.* Jun 15 2008;167(12):1446-1452.

51. Skopp NA, Trofimovich L, Grimes J, Oetjen-Gerdes L, Gahm GA. Relations between suicide and traumatic brain injury, psychiatric diagnoses, and relationship problems, active component, U.S. Armed Forces, 2001-2009. *Msmr.* Feb 2012;19(2):7-11.

52. Theeler BJ, Flynn FG, Erickson JC. Headaches after concussion in US soldiers returning from Iraq or Afghanistan. *Headache.* Sep 2010;50(8):1262-1272.

53. Theeler BJ, Flynn FG, Erickson JC. Chronic Daily Headache in U.S. Soldiers After Concussion. *Headache.* 2012;52(5):732-738.

54. Vanderploeg RD, Belanger HG, Curtiss G. Mild traumatic brain injury and posttraumatic stress disorder and their associations with health symptoms. *Arch Phys Med Rehabil.* Jul 2009;90(7):1084-1093.

55. Vanderploeg RD, Curtiss G, Belanger HG. Long-term neuropsychological outcomes following mild traumatic brain injury. *J Int Neuropsychol Soc.* May 2005;11(3):228-236.

56. Vanderploeg RD, Curtiss G, Duchnick JJ, Luis CA. Demographic, medical, and psychiatric factors in work and marital status after mild head injury. *J Head Trauma Rehabil.* Mar-Apr 2003;18(2):148-163.

57. Vasterling JJ, Brailey K, Proctor SP, Kane R, Heeren T, Franz M. Neuropsychological outcomes of mild traumatic brain injury, post-traumatic stress disorder and depression in Iraq-deployed US Army soldiers. *Br J Psychiatry.* Sep 2012;201:186-192.

58. Wilk JE, Herrell RK, Wynn GH, Riviere LA, Hoge CW. Mild traumatic brain injury (concussion), posttraumatic stress disorder, and depression in U.S. soldiers involved in combat deployments: association with postdeployment symptoms. *Psychosom Med.* Apr 2012;74(3):249-257.

59. Wilk JE, Thomas JL, McGurk DM, Riviere LA, Castro CA, Hoge CW. Mild traumatic brain injury (concussion) during combat: lack of association of blast mechanism with persistent postconcussive symptoms. *J Head Trauma Rehabil.* Jan-Feb 2010;25(1):9-14.

60. Yurkiewicz IR, Lappan CM, Neely ET, et al. Outcomes from a US military neurology and traumatic brain injury telemedicine program. *Neurology.* Sep 18 2012;79(12):1237-1243.

# APPENDIX E. RESULTS OF INCLUDED STUDIES

## Cognitive Functioning

### Table 1a. Language abilities and general fund of verbal knowledge measures in studies of U.S. Veterans and members of the U.S. military with mild TBI

| Author, year | Comparison group description | Outcome measure | Subscale or test component | mTBI group Mean (SD) | Comparison group Mean (SD) | p value for comparison | Magnitude of effect |
|---|---|---|---|---|---|---|---|
| Nelson, Hoelzle, Doane, et al., 2012[29] | Axis I disorder | WTAR scaled score | --- | 106.7 (10.1) | 105.4 (5.7) | "NS" | NR |
| | | WAIS-III | Information scaled score | 12.8 (1.7) | 11.8 (2.1) | "NS" | NR |
| | Forensic context | WAIS-III | Information scaled score | 11.97 (1.92) | 11.58 (1.82) | "NS" | NR |
| Cooper, Chau, Armistead-Jehle, et al., 2012[16] | Blast exposed | RBANS | Language | 97.43 (12.42) | 92.81 (14.10) | p = 0.187 | NR |
| Drag, Spencer, Walker, et al., 2012[20] | LOC and/or PTA | Shipley Institute of Living Scale | Vocabulary Subtest | 49.15 (7.50) | 49.15 (6.20) | NR | NR |
| Gordon, Fitzpatrick, Hilsabeck, 2011[22] | Mental Health Diagnosis other than PTSD | WTAR | --- | 96.8 (10.8) | 101.7 (12.3) | NR | NR |
| Gordon, Fitzpatrick, Hilsabeck, 2011[22] | PTSD Diagnosis | WTAR | --- | 96.8 (10.8) | 99.0 (11.2) | NR | NR |
| Belanger, Kretzmer, Venderploeg, & French, 2010[10] | Same population with moderate/severe TBI | WTAR | Estimated Full Scale IQ (FSIQ) | 98.3 (9.3) | 97.6 (9.1) | p = .67 | NR |
| Belanger, Kretzmer, Yoash-Gantz, Pickett, & Tupler, 2009[11] | Same population with moderate/severe TBI | WTAR | Estimated Full Scale IQ (FSIQ) | 98.1 (14.6) | 96.1 (12.8) | p = .35 | NR |
| Cooper, Mercado-Couch, Critchfield, et al., 2010[18] | Same population without mTBI | RBANS | Language | 92.90 (15.586) | 93.66 (11.873) | p = 0.732 | NR |
| Nelson, Hoelzle, McGuire, et al., 2010[30] | Same population without mTBI; none with poor effort | WAIS-III | Information scaled score | 12.21 (2.01) | 12.26 (2.25) | "NS" | d = .22 |
| Nelson, Hoelzle, Doane, et al., 2012[29] | Same population without mTBI; none have Axis I | WAIS-III | Information scaled score | 12.8 (1.7) | 11.9 (2.6) | "NS" | NR |
| | | WTAR | scaled score | 106.7 (10.1) | 106.0 (9.2) | "NS" | NR |

## Table 1b. Visuospatial function in studies of U.S. Veterans and members of the U.S. military with mild TBI

| Author, year | Comparison group description | Outcome measure | Subscale or test component | mTBI group Mean (SD) | Comparison group Mean (SD) | p value for comparison | Magnitude of effect |
|---|---|---|---|---|---|---|---|
| Spencer, et al., 2010[36] | NA | RCFT | Figure Copy | 33.6 (2.9) | NA | NA | NA |
| | | | Figure Orientation | 3.6 (1.7) | NA | NA | NA |
| | | | Time to Copy | 158.7 (63.5) | NA | NA | NA |
| Cooper, Mercado-Couch, Critchfield, et al., 2010[18] | Same population without mTBI | RBANS | Visuospatial/Constructional | 104.06 (13.382) | 109.29 (10.47) | p = 0.007 | NR |
| Nelson, Hoelzle, Doane, et al., 2012[29] | Same population without mTBI; none have Axis I | RCFT | Figure Copy | 31.3 (3.2) | 32.0 (2.1) | "NS" | NR |
| | | WAIS-III | Block Design scaled score | 12.2 (2.6) | 13.0 (2.9) | "NS" | NR |
| Nelson, Hoelzle, Doane, et al., 2012[29] | Axis I disorder | RCFT | Figure Copy | 31.3 (3.2) | 31.5 (3.0) | "NS" | NR |
| | | WAIS-III | Block Design scaled score | 12.2 (2.6) | 12.2 (3.1) | "NS" | NR |
| Cooper, Chau, Armistead-Jehle, et al., 2012[16] | Blast exposed | RBANS | Visuospatial/Constructional | 112.11 (9.70) | 108.09 (11.80) | p = 0.159 | NR |
| Drag, Spencer, Walker, et al., 2012[20] | HADS Anxiety | Visual Organization/Processing Factor | --- | NR | NR | p > .05 | r = -.12 |
| | HADS Depression | Visual Organization/Processing Factor | --- | NR | NR | p < .001 | r = -.25 |
| | LOC and/or PTA | Visual Organization/Processing Factor | --- | 49.08 (9.98) | 50.46 (10.12) | p = .30 | NR |
| | | RCFT | Figure Copy | 33.72 (2.64) | 33.78 (2.38) | NR | NR |
| | | | Organization | 3.64 (1.74) | 3.99 (1.81) | NR | NR |
| | | | Time to Copy | 170.51 (63.07) | 166.17 (74.91) | NR | NR |
| Gordon, Fitzpatrick, Hilsabeck, 2011[22] | Mental Health Diagnosis other than PTSD | RCFT | Figure Copy | 32.6 (4.9) | 32.7 (4.7) | NR | NR |
| Drag, Spencer, Walker, et al., 2012[20] | PCL-M score | Visual Organization/Processing Factor | --- | NR | NR | p < .05 | r = -.18 |
| Gordon, Fitzpatrick, Hilsabeck, 2011[22] | PTSD Diagnosis | RCFT | Figure Copy | 32.6 (4.9) | 32.1 (6.0) | NR | NR |
| Spencer et al., 2010[36] | Self-reported slowed thinking/organization | RCFT | Figure Copy | NR | NR | "NS" | r = -.13 |
| | | | Figure Orientation | NR | NR | "NS" | r = -.02 |
| | | | Time to Copy | NR | NR | "NS" | r = -.14 |
| Drag, Spencer, Walker, et al., 2012[20] | Service connected | Visual Organization/Processing Factor | --- | NR | NR | p = .57 | NR |

## Table 1c. Memory functioning in studies of U.S. Veterans and members of the U.S. military with mild TBI

| Author, year | Comparison group description | Outcome measure | Subscale or test component | mTBI group Mean (SD) or Median (IQR) | Comparison group Mean (SD) or Median (IQR) | p value for comparison | Magnitude of effect |
|---|---|---|---|---|---|---|---|
| Nelson, Hoelzle, Doane, et al., 2012[29] | Axis I disorder | CVLT-II | Long Delay Free Recall z-score | 0.5 (0.9) | -0.1 (1.1) | "Significant" | NR |
| | | | Trials 1-5 z-score | 0.6 (0.9) | 0.1 (1.0) | "NS" | NR |
| | | RCFT | Delayed Recall z-score | -0.1 (1.3) | -0.5 (.98) | "NS" | NR |
| Belanger, Kretzmer, Yoash-Gantz, Pickett, & Tupler, 2009[11] | Blast exposure | BVMT-R | Delayed Recall t score | 48.6 (12.8) | 50.7 (10.7) | "NS" | NR |
| | | | Total Recall t score | 45.2 (12.3) | 50.1 (10.1) | "NS" | NR |
| | | CVLT-II | Long Delay Free Recall t-score | 48.3 (9.1) | 50.5 (11.4) | p = .38 | NR |
| | | | Total Trials 1-5 t-score | 52.8 (10.5) | 54.0 (8.1) | p = .38 | NR |
| Cooper, Chau, Armistead-Jehle, et al., 2012[16] | Blast exposure | RBANS | Immediate Memory | 91.70 (11.0) | 91.81 (15.67) | P = 0.994 | NR |
| | | | Delayed Memory | 96.96 (16.59) | 95.12 (16.04) | P = 0.664 | NR |
| Nelson, Hoelzle, McGuire, et al., 2010[30] | Forensic context | CVLT-II | Long Delay Free Recall z-score | 0.03 (0.99) | -0.73 (1.12) | "NS" | NR |
| | | | Trials 1-5 t-score | 52.82 (8.61) | 46.33 (9.23) | "NS" | NR |
| Drag, Spencer, Walker, et al., 2012[20] | HADS Anxiety | Memory Factor | --- | NR | NR | p < .001 | r = -.29 |
| Drag, Spencer, Walker, et al., 2012[20] | HADS Depression | Memory Factor | --- | NR | NR | p > .05 | r = -.15 |
| Drag, Spencer, Walker, et al., 2012[20] | LOC and/or PTA | Memory Factor | --- | 49.22 (9.89) | 49.61 (10.36) | NR | NR |
| | | RBANS | Story Memory Immediate Recall | 44.99 (10.19) | 48.10 (10.36) | NR | NR |
| | | | Story Memory Delayed Recall | 45.41 (10.49) | 44.98 (10.71) | NR | NR |
| | | RCFT | Immediate Recall | 44.43 (12.72) | 44.50 (13.65) | NR | NR |
| Gordon, Fitzpatrick, Hilsabeck, 2011[22] | Mental Health Diagnosis other than PTSD | CVLT-II | Long Delay Free Recall | 8.9 (3.7) | 8.9 (3.9) | NR | NR |
| | | | Short Delay Free Recall | 8.3 (3.5) | 8.6 (3.9) | NR | NR |
| | | CVLT-II | Total Trials 1-5 | 43.7 (12.0) | 44.6 (13.7) | NR | NR |
| | | RCFT | Immediate Recall | 16.4 (7.7) | 17.4 (7.2) | NR | NR |
| | | | Delayed Recall | 16.0 (7.9) | 17.4 (7.2) | NR | NR |

# Complications of Mild Traumatic Brain Injury in Veterans and Military Personnel: A Systematic Review

| Author, year | Comparison group description | Outcome measure | Subscale or test component | mTBI group Mean (SD) or Median (IQR) | Comparison group Mean (SD) or Median (IQR) | p value for comparison | Magnitude of effect |
|---|---|---|---|---|---|---|---|
| Spencer, et al., 2010[36] | No comparison group | RBANS | Story Memory Immediate Recall | 17.2 (3.4) | NA | NA | NA |
| | | | Story Memory Delayed Recall | 8.4 (2.3) | NA | NA | NA |
| | | RCFT | Immediate Recall | 19.9 (6.2) | NA | NA | NA |
| | | | MSP subtest | Baseline: 51 (43-53) ≤72 hours: 44 (38.5-51) | Baseline: 50 (45-55) ≤72 hours: 50 (44-56) | Baseline: p =.57 ≤72 hours: p <.001 | NR |
| Drag, Spencer, Walker, et al., 2012[20] | PCL-M score | Memory Factor | --- | NR | NR | p < .05 | r = -.34 |
| Gordon, Fitzpatrick, Hilsabeck, 2011[22] | PTSD Diagnosis | CVLT-II | Long Delay Free Recall | 8.9 (3.7) | 7.6 (3.2) | NR | NR |
| | | | Short Delay Free Recall | 8.3 (3.5) | 7.0 (3.4) | NR | NR |
| | | | Total Trials 1-5 | 43.7 (12.0) | 38.7 (11.1) | NR | NR |
| | | RCFT | Immediate Recall | 16.4 (7.7) | 15.7 (8.5) | NR | NR |
| | | | Delayed Recall | 16.0 (7.9) | 16.1 (7.1) | NR | NR |
| Nelson, Hoelzle, McGuire, et al., 2010[30] | Same population of research participants, none with poor effort | CVLT-II | Long Delay Free Recall z-score | 0.27 (0.91) | 0.45 (0.81) | "NS" | d = 0.21 |
| | | | Trials 1-5 t-score | 54.43 (8.95) | 57.16 (8.04) | "NS" | d = 0.32 |
| Belanger, Kretzmer, Yoash-Gantz, Pickett, & Tupler, 2009[11] | Same population with moderate/ severe TBI | BVMT-R | Delayed Recall | NR | NR | "NS" | NR |
| | | BVMT-R | Total Recall | NR | NR | "NS" | NR |
| | | CVLT-II | Long Delay Free Recall | NR | NR | p < .05 | NR |
| | | | Total Trials 1-5 | NR | NR | p < .01 | NR |
| Schiehser, Delis, Filoteo, et al., 2011[35] | Same population with moderate/ severe TBI | Memory Composite Score | --- | 9.0 (2.4) | 7.7 (2.8) | p = .04 | NR |
| Coldren, Russell, Parish, et al., 2012[15] | Same population without mTBI; with minor traumatic injuries not involving the head and noninjured volunteers from same population | ANAM | CDD subtest | Baseline: 42.5 (36.5-50) 5+ days: 49.5 (40-56) 10+ days: 49.5 (40.1-53.1) | Baseline: 44 (37-52) 5+ days: 50.3 (44.1-57.8) 10+ days: 50.3 (44.1-57.8) | Baseline: p = 0.47 5+ days: p = 0.07 10+ days: p = 0.17 | NR |
| | | | MSP subtest | Baseline: 51 (43-53) 5+ days: 50.5 (44-58) 10+ days: 51.8 (43.5-57.9) | Baseline: 52 (44.5-57.8) 5+ days: 51.5 (44.5-57.6) 10+ days: 51.5 (44.5-57.6) | Baseline: p = 0.29 5+ days: p = 0.47 10+ days: p = 0.77 | NR |
| Cooper, Mercado-Couch, Critchfield, et al., 2010[18] | Same population without TBI | RBANS | Immediate Memory | 95.14 (14.181) | 96.49 (14.445) | p = .589 | NR |

| Author, year | Comparison group description | Outcome measure | Subscale or test component | mTBI group Mean (SD) or Median (IQR) | Comparison group Mean (SD) or Median (IQR) | p value for comparison | Magnitude of effect |
|---|---|---|---|---|---|---|---|
| Kelly, Coldren, Parish, et al., 2012[24] | Same population without mTBI; with minor traumatic injuries not involving the head and noninjured volunteers from same population | ANAM | CDD subtest | Baseline: 42.5 (35-50) ≤ 72 hours: 42 (35-49.5) | Baseline: 45 (38-52) ≤ 72 hours: 44.75 (39-51) | Baseline: p = .20 ≤ 72 hours: p = .04 | NR |
| Nelson, Hoelzle, Doane, et al., 2012[29] | Same population without mTBI; none have Axis I | CVLT-II | Long Delay Free Recall z-score | 0.5 (0.9) | 0.6 (0.8) | "NS" | NR |
| | | | Trials 1-5 z-score | 0.6 (0.9) | 0.8 (0.8) | "NS" | NR |
| | | RCFT | Delayed Recall z-score | -0.1 (1.3) | -0.3 (1.3) | "NS" | NR |
| | | | Delayed Memory | 96.48 (12.998) | 100.42 (12.854) | p = 0.072 | NR |
| Spencer et al., 2010[36] | Self-reported memory deficits | RBANS | Story Memory Immediate Recall | NR | NR | "NS" | r = -.05 |
| | | | Story Memory Delayed Recall | NR | NR | p < .05 | r = -.20 |
| | | RCFT | Immediate Recall | NR | NR | "NS" | r = .08 |
| Drag, Spencer, Walker, et al., 2012[20] | Service connected | Memory Factor | ---- | NR | NR | p = .17 | NR |

83

## Table 1d. Attention/concentration measures in studies of U.S. Veterans and members of the U.S. military with mTBI

| Author, year | Comparison group description | Outcome measure | Subscale or test component | mTBI group Mean (SD) or Median (IQR) | Comparison group Mean (SD) or Median (IQR) | p value for comparison | Magnitude of effect |
|---|---|---|---|---|---|---|---|
| Nelson, Hoelzle, Doane, et al., 2012[29] | Axis I disorder | WAIS-III | Digit Span scaled score | 9.9 (2.8) | 9.9 (2.1) | "NS" | NR |
| | Forensic context | WAIS-III | Digit Span scaled score | 9.61 (2.55) | 8.42 (2.77) | "NS" | NR |
| Cooper, Chau, Armistead-Jehle, et al., 2012[16] | Blast exposure | RBANS | Attention | 98.89 (16.64) | 94.78 (14.51) | p = 0.311 | NA |
| Drag, Spencer, Walker, et al., 2012[20] | HADS Anxiety | Verbal Attention Factor | -- | NR | NR | p < .05 | r = -.24 |
| | | Visual Attention Factor | -- | NR | NR | p > .05 | r = -.12 |
| | HADS Depression | Verbal Attention Factor | -- | NR | NR | p < .05 | r = -.24 |
| | | Visual Attention Factor | -- | NR | NR | p > .05 | r = -.13 |
| | LOC and/or PTA | Verbal Attention Factor | -- | 49.69 (10.91) | 49.87 (9.69) | p = .91 | NR |
| | | Visual Attention Factor | -- | 50.67 (9.61) | 49.61 (10.36) | p = .50 | NR |
| | LOC and/or PTA | WAIS-IV | Digit Sequencing | 9.30 (2.76) | 9.41 (2.27) | NR | NR |
| | | | Digit Span Backward | 9.23 (2.54) | 8.92 (2.18) | NR | NR |
| | | | Digits Forward | 8.39 (2.63) | 8.64 (2.70) | NR | NR |
| Spencer et al., 2010[36] | No comparison group | WAIS-IV | Digit Sequencing | 8.0 (1.9) | NA | NA | NA |
| | | | Digits Backward | 7.8 (2.1) | NA | NA | NA |
| | | | Digits Forward | 9.6 (2.1) | NA | NA | NA |
| Drag, Spencer, Walker, et al., 2012[20] | PCL-M score | Verbal Attention Factor | -- | NR | NR | p < .05 | r = -.21 |
| | | Visual Attention Factor | -- | NR | NR | p < .05 | r = -.20 |
| | | | Digit Span scaled score | 9.9 (2.8) | 10.9 (2.4) | "NS" | NR |
| Coldren, Russell, Parish, et al., 2012[15] | Same population without mTBI; with minor traumatic injuries not involving the head and noninjured volunteers from same population | ANAM | Mathematical Processing (MTH) subtest | Baseline: 51 (42-57.3)<br><br>5+ days: 50.5 (43-56)<br><br>10+ days: 50.8 (46.3-55.8) | Baseline: 50 (42-55)<br><br>5+ days: 52 (44-59.8)<br><br>10+ days: 52 (44-59.8) | Baseline: p = 0.71<br><br>5+ days: p = 0.29<br><br>10+ days: p = 0.51 | NR |
| Cooper, Mercado-Couch, Critchfield, et al., 2010[18] | Same population without mTBI | RBANS | Attention | 84.06 (15.013) | 89.74 (14.898) | p = 0.026 | NR |

| Author, year | Comparison group description | Outcome measure | Subscale or test component | mTBI group Mean (SD) or Median (IQR) | Comparison group Mean (SD) or Median (IQR) | p value for comparison | Magnitude of effect |
|---|---|---|---|---|---|---|---|
| Kelly, Coldren, Parish, et al., 2012[24] | Same population without mTBI; with minor traumatic injuries not involving the head and noninjured volunteers from same population | ANAM | Mathematical Processing (MTH) subtest | Baseline: 47 (42-57) / ≤72 hours: 46.7 (40.5-52.5) | Baseline: 52 (42-55) / ≤72 hours: 50 (44-56.6) | Baseline: p = .57 / ≤72 hours: p = .03 | NR |
| Nelson, Hoelzle, McGuire, et al., 2010[30] | Same population without mTBI; none with poor effort | WAIS-III | Digit Span scaled score | 10.50 (2.29) | 10.65 (2.37) | "NS" | d = .06 |
| Spencer, et al., 2010[36] | Self-reported attention deficits | WAIS-IV | Digit Sequencing | NR | NR | "NS" | r = -.15 |
| | | | Digits Backward | NR | NR | "NS" | r = -.11 |
| | | | Digits Forward | NR | NR | "NS" | r = -.15 |
| | | | Digit Sequencing | NR | NR | "NS" | r = .00 |
| | | | Digits Backward | NR | NR | "NS" | r = -.14 |
| Drag, Spencer, Walker, et al., 2012[20] | Service connected | | Verbal Attention Factor | --- | NR | p = .42 | NR |
| | | | Visual Attention Factor | --- | NR | p = .17 | NR |

## Table 1e. Cognitive processing speed in studies of U.S. Veterans and members of the U.S. military with mild TBI

| Author, year | Comparison group description | Outcome measure | Subscale or test component | mTBI group Mean (SD) or Median (IQR) | Comparison group Mean (SD) or Median (IQR) | p value for comparison | Magnitude of effect |
|---|---|---|---|---|---|---|---|
| Nelson, Hoelzle, Doane, et al., 2012[29] | Axis I disorder | Stroop Color and Word Test | Color t-score | 49.5 (6.9) | 45.8 (7.8) | "NS" | NR |
| | | | Word t-score | 49.4 (9.8) | 46.2 (8.6) | "NS" | NR |
| | | Trail Making Test | Part A t-score | 50.0 (11.7) | 50.5 (9.7) | "NS" | NR |
| | | WAIS-III | Digit Symbol Coding scaled score | 10.9 (2.0) | 9.8 (2.4) | "NS" | NR |
| Belanger, Kretzmer, Yoash-Gantz, Pickett, & Tupler, 2009[11] | Blast exposure | Trail Making Test | Part A t-score | 45.8 (14.8) | 46.2 (11.6) | all p values > .10 | NR |
| | | WAIS-III | Digit Symbol Coding scaled score | 8.3 (2.7) | 8.9 (2.5) | all p values > .10 | NR |

| Author, year | Comparison group description | Outcome measure | Subscale or test component | mTBI group Mean (SD) or Median (IQR) | Comparison group Mean (SD) or Median (IQR) | p value for comparison | Magnitude of effect |
|---|---|---|---|---|---|---|---|
| Nelson, Hoelzle, McGuire, et al., 2010[30] | Forensic context | Stroop Color and Word Test | Color t-score | 45.29 (8.60) | 40.04 (7.00) | "NS" | NR |
|  |  |  | Word t-score | 45.47 (9.01) | 39.12 (7.54) | "NS" | NR |
|  |  | Trail Making Test | Part A t-score | 48.71 (10.44) | 39.96 (9.78) | "Significant" | NR |
|  |  | WAIS-III | Digit Symbol Coding scaled score | 9.92 (2.53) | 7.12 (2.53) | "Significant" | NR |
| Drag, Spencer, Walker, et al., 2012[20] | LOC and/or PTA | Trail Making Test | Part A | 48.93 (10.83) | 47.99 (11.04) | NR | NR |
| Gordon, Fitzpatrick, Hilsabeck, 2011[22] | Mental Health Diagnosis other than PTSD | Stroop Color & Word Test | Color | 58.8 (12.1) | 54.1 (11.2) | NR | NR |
|  |  |  | Word | 76.2 (16.5) | 77.0 (17.7) | NR | NR |
|  |  | Trail Making Test | Part A | 41.8 (15.8) | 41.9 (19.1) | NR | NR |
| Spencer et al., 2010[36] | No comparison group | Trail Making Test | Part A | 29.6 (13.1) | NA | NA | NA |
|  |  |  | Procedural Reaction Time (PRT) subtest | Baseline: 52 (43-53) ≤72 hours: 46 (34.5-54.5) | Baseline: 50 (47-58) ≤72 hours: 52.5 (46.5-59) | Baseline: p = .60 ≤72 hours: p < .001 | NR |
|  |  |  | Simple Reaction Time (SRT) subtest | Baseline: 53 (48-55) ≤72 hours: 44.5 (34.5-52) | Baseline: 52 (47-55) ≤72 hours: 52 (47-55.5) | Baseline: p = .24 ≤72 hours: p < .001 | NR |
| Gordon, Fitzpatrick, Hilsabeck, 2011[22] | PTSD Diagnosis | Stroop Color & Word Test | Color | 58.8 (12.1) | 60.8 (15.3) | NR | NR |
|  |  |  | Word | 76.2 (16.5) | 79.6 (18.2) | NR | NR |
|  |  | Trail Making Test | Part A | 41.8 (15.8) | 40.1 (15.0) | NR | NR |
| Coldren, Russell, Parish, et al., 2012[15] | Same population without mTBI; with minor traumatic injuries not involving the head and noninjured volunteers from same population | ANAM | Code Substitution (CDS) subtest | Baseline: 46 (39.5-48.5) 5+ days: 52.5 (46.5-58) 10+ days: 53 (47-60) | Baseline: 48 (43-55) 5+ days: 57 (50-63) 10+ days: 57 (50-63) | Baseline: p = 0.04 5+ days: p = 0.03 10+ days: p = 0.14 | NR |
|  |  |  | Procedural Reaction Time (PRT) subtest | Baseline: 52 (43-57) 5+ days: 52 (44.5-58.5) 10+ days: 48.8 (42-62.1) | Baseline: 52 (47-58) 5+ days: 54 (47-62.5) 10+ days: 54 (47-62.5) | Baseline: p = 0.77 5+ days: p = 0.13 10+ days: p = 0.20 | NR |
|  |  |  | Simple Reaction Time (SRT) subtest | Baseline: 53 (52-55) 5+ days: 54 (48-56.5) 10+ days: 54.5 (46.6-57.6) | Baseline: 52 (47-58) 5+ days: 53.5 (48.8-56.5) 10+ days: 53.5 (48.8-56.5) | Baseline: p = .23 5+ days: p = .97 10+ days: p = .71 | NR |
| Kelly, Coldren, Parish, et al., 2012[24] | Same population without mTBI; with minor traumatic injuries not involving the head and noninjured volunteers from same population | ANAM | Code Substitution (CDS) subtest | Baseline: 44 (37-50) ≤72 hours: 44 (38.5-51) | - Baseline: 48 (43-55) ≤72 hours: 52 (45-57) | Baseline: p = .02 ≤72 hours: p < .001 | NR |

**Complications of Mild Traumatic Brain Injury in Veterans and Military Personnel: A Systematic Review**

| Author, year | Comparison group description | Outcome measure | Subscale or test component | mTBI group Mean (SD) or Median (IQR) | Comparison group Mean (SD) or Median (IQR) | p value for comparison | Magnitude of effect |
|---|---|---|---|---|---|---|---|
| Nelson, Hoelzle, McGuire, et al., 2010[30] | Same population without mTBI; none with poor effort | Stroop Color and Word Test | Color t-score | 46.00 (8.88) | 47.26 (6.90) | "NS" | d = 0.16 |
| | | | Word t-score | 46.29 (9.10) | 48.58 (8.64) | "NS" | d = 0.26 |
| | | Trail Making Test | Part A t-score | 48.89 (9.89) | 49.61 (11.66) | "NS" | d = 0.10 |
| | | WAIS-III | Digit Symbol Coding scaled score | 10.46 (2.52) | 10.35 (2.47) | "NS" | d = 0.04 |
| Nelson, Hoelzle, Doane, et al., 2012[29] | Same population without mTBI; none have Axis I | Stroop Color and Word Test | Color t-score | 49.5 (6.9) | 48.9 (6.7) | "NS" | NR |
| Swick, Honzel, Larsen, et al., 2012[37] | Same population without mTBI; participants had PTSD | Reaction time on a Go/NoGo task | --- | NR | NR | p > .7 | NR |
| Belanger, Kretzmer, Yoash-Gantz, Pickett, & Tupler, 2009[11] | Same population with moderate/severe TBI | Trail Making Test | Part A | NR | NR | all p values > .10 | NR |
| | | WAIS-III | Digit Symbol Coding | NR | NR | all p values > .10 | NR |
| | | | Word t-score | 49.4 (9.8) | 48.3 (6.6) | "NS" | NR |
| | | Trail Making Test | Part A t-score | 50.0 (11.7) | 51.8 (12.1) | "NS" | NR |
| | | WAIS-III | Digit Symbol Coding scaled score | 10.9 (2.0) | 11.1 (2.7) | "NS" | NR |
| Spencer, et al., 2010[36] | Self-reported attention deficits | Trail Making Test | Part A | NR | NR | "NS" | r = -.03 |
| Spencer, et al., 2010[36] | Self-reported slowed thinking/organization | Trail Making Test | Part A | NR | NR | "NS" | r = -.09 |

**Table 1f. Executive functioning in studies of U.S. Veterans and members of the U.S. military with mild TBI**

| Author, year | Comparison group description | Outcome measure | Subscale or test component | mTBI group Mean (SD) | Comparison group Mean (SD) | p value for comparison | Magnitude of effect |
|---|---|---|---|---|---|---|---|
| Belanger, Kretzmer, Yoash-Gantz, Pickett, & Tupler, 2009[11] | Blast exposure | Trail Making Test | Part B t-score | 49.1 (15.0) | 45.6 (9.4) | all p values > .10 | NR |
| | Same population with moderate/severe TBI | Trail Making Test | Part B | NR | NR | all p values > .10 | NR |
| Drag, Spencer, Walker, et al., 2012[20] | LOC and/or PTA | Trail Making Test | Part B t-score | 49.96 (8.35) | 48.80 (8.65) | NR | NR |
| Gordon, Fitzpatrick, Hilsabeck, 2011[22] | Mental Health Diagnosis other than PTSD | Stroop Color & Word Test | Color Word | 32.9 (7.9) | 30.3 (9.0) | NR | NR |
| | | Trail Making Test | Part B | 93.0 (38.8) | 106.1 (73.2) | NR | NR |
| | PTSD Diagnosis | Stroop Color & Word Test | Color Word | 32.9 (7.9) | 30.5 (8.5) | NR | NR |
| | | Trail Making Test | Part B | 93.0 (38.8) | 95.2 (34.5) | NR | NR |
| Nelson, Hoelzle, Doane, et al., 2012[29] | Axis I disorder | COWA t-score | -- | 46.4 (11.0) | 42.7 (9.5) | "NS" | NR |
| | | Stroop Color and Word Test | Color-Word t-score | 51.1 (9.5) | 48.3 (9.5) | "NS" | NR |
| | | Trail Making Test | Part B t-score | 51.0 (12.1) | 48.4 (10.8) | "NS" | NR |
| | Same population without mTBI; none have Axis I | COWA t-score | -- | 46.4 (11.0) | 48.9 (9.7) | "NS" | NR |
| | | Stroop Color and Word Test | Color-Word t-score | 51.1 (9.5) | 52.6 (7.0) | "NS" | NR |
| | | Trail Making Test | Part B t-score | 51.0 (12.1) | 53.6 (7.5) | "NS" | NR |
| Nelson, Hoelzle, McGuire, et al., 2010[30] | Forensic context | COWA t-score | -- | 44.79 (10.43) | 42.83 (8.52) | "NS" | NR |
| | | Stroop Color and Word Test | Color-Word t-score | 46.95 (9.09) | 43.78 (8.10) | "NS" | NR |
| | | Trail Making Test | Part B t-score | 51.45 (10.25) | 44.71 (10.22) | "NS" | NR |
| | Same population without mTBI; none with poor effort | COWA t-score | | 47.04 (8.94) | 46.97 (9.69) | "NS" | d = 0.01 |
| | | Stroop Color and Word Test | Color-Word t-score | 48.86 (9.35) | 50.52 (9.22) | "NS" | d = 0.18 |
| | | Trail Making Test | Part B t-score | 52.21 (10.20) | 52.77 (5.83) | NS | d = 0.07 |
| Schiehser, Delis, Filoteo, et al., 2011[35] | Same population with moderate/severe TBI | Executive Function Composite Score | -- | 10.4 (2.2) | 9.5 (3.0) | p = .13 | NR |
| Spencer, et al., 2010[36] | None | Trail Making Test | Part B | 72.8 (34.8) | NA | NA | NA |
| | Self-reported attention deficits | Trail Making Test | Part B | NR | NR | "NS" | r = -.01 |
| | Self-reported slowed thinking/organization | Trail Making Test | Part B | NR | NR | "NS" | r = -.01 |

Table 1g. Effort and motivation measures in a study of U.S. Veterans with mild TBI evaluated in a research versus forensic context

| Author, year | Outcome measure | Portion or subscale | Research context Mean (SD) | Forensic context Mean (SD) | p value for comparison | Magnitude of effect |
|---|---|---|---|---|---|---|
| Nelson, Hoelzle, McGuire, et al., 2010[30] | CVLT-II | Forced Choice | 15.87 (0.41) | 15.50 (1.18) | "NS" | NR |
| | Effort Failures raw score | --- | 0.32 (0.58) | 1.17 (0.87) | "Significant" | NR |
| | Rey FIT | Combination | 28.84 (2.06) | 26.13 (3.72) | "Significant" | NR |
| | VSVT | Easy Items | 23.90 (0.31) | 22.92 (2.00) | "Significant" | NR |
| | | Difficult Items | 22.11 (2.87) | 15.63 (6.25) | "Significant" | NR |
| | | Total Items | 46.00 (3.08) | 38.54 (7.43) | "Significant" | NR |
| | WAIS-III | Reliable Digit Span | 9.63 (1.98) | 8.38 (1.71) | "NS" | NR |

## Table 1h. Total and cross-domain composite scores in studies of U.S. Veterans and members of the U.S. military with mild TBI

| Author, year | Comparison group description | Outcome measure | Subscale or test component | mTBI group Mean (SD) | Comparison group Mean (SD) | p value for comparison | Magnitude of effect |
|---|---|---|---|---|---|---|---|
| Cooper, Chau, Armistead-Jehle, et al., 2012[16] | Blast exposure | RBANS | Total Score | 98.61 (9.33) | 94.88 (12.92) | p = 0.211 | NR |
| Cooper, Mercado-Couch, Critchfield, et al., 2010[18] | Same population without mTBI | RBANS | Total Score | 92.16 (11.932) | 96.71 (11.672) | p = 0.023 | NR |
| Nelson, Hoelzle, McGuire, et al., 2010[30] | Same population without mTBI; none with poor effort | Overall Test Battery Mean z-score | -- | 0.00 (0.55) | 0.11 (0.42) | "NS" | d = 0.22 |
| Nelson, Hoelzle, Doane, et al., 2012[29] | Same population without mTBI; none have Axis I | Overall Test Battery Mean z-score | -- | 0.14 (0.69) | 0.26 (0.38) | "NS" | d = .23 |
| Schiehser, Delis, Filoteo, et al., 2011[35] | Same population with moderate/severe TBI | Attention/Processing Speed Composite Score | -- | 9.8 (1.9) | 8.5 (2.0) | p < .01 | NR |
| Nelson, Hoelzle, Doane, et al., 2012[29] | Axis I disorder | Overall Test Battery Mean z-score | -- | 0.14 (0.69) | -.14 (.45) | "NS" | NR |
| Nelson, Hoelzle, McGuire, et al., 2010[30] | Forensic context | Overall Test Battery Mean z-score | -- | -0.15 (0.55) | -0.75 (0.52) | "Significant" | NR |
| Ruff, Ruff, & Wang, 2009[34] | Headache intervention involving sleep hygiene, Prazosin, headache and pain education, and group therapy | MOCA | -- | 24.50 (.49) | 28.60 (.59) | p < .001 | NR |
| Ruff, Riechers, Wang, et al., 2012[32] | LOC | MOCA | -- | 28.9 (.32) | 25.1 (.18) | p < .001 | NR |
| Gordon, Fitzpatrick, Hilsabeck, 2011[22] | Mental Health Diagnosis other than PTSD | WAIS-III (73 participants administered); WAIS-IV (9 participants administered) | WAIS-III Vocabulary, Information, Matrix Reasoning, Block Design Subscales; WAIS-IV: all subtests | 97.4 (11.0) | 100.2 (15.4) | NR | NR |
| Ruff, Ruff, & Wang, 2008[33] | Positive neurological and/ or neuropsychological findings | Number of blast exposures associated with LOC or AOC | -- | 2.65 (.18) | 4.42 (.23) | p < .001 | NR |
| | | Number of blast exposures associated with LOC only | -- | 1.46 (.09) | 3.91 (.20) | p < .001 | NR |
| Gordon, Fitzpatrick, Hilsabeck, 2011[22] | PTSD Diagnosis | WAIS-III (73 participants administered); WAIS-IV: (9 participants administered) | WAIS-III Vocabulary, Information, Matrix Reasoning, Block Design Subscales; WAIS-IV: all subtests | 97.4 (11.0) | 95.6 (13.3) | NR | NR |

## Table 1i. Self-reported cognitive deficits in studies of U.S. Veterans and members of the U.S. military with mild TBI

| Author, year | Comparison group description | Outcome measure | Subscale or test component | mTBI group Mean (SD) | Comparison group Mean (SD) | p value for comparison | Magnitude of effect |
|---|---|---|---|---|---|---|---|
| Kennedy, Cullen, Amador, et al., 2010[25] | At least one additional AIS code | NSI | Cognitive Cluster | 10.01 (4.90) | 6.88 (5.25) | p < 0.001 | NR |
| | | | Concentration | 2.16 (1.17) | 1.40 (1.32) | p < 0.001 | NR |
| | | | Decision-Making | 1.74 (1.22) | 1.04 (1.15) | p < 0.001 | NR |
| | | | Memory | 2.36 (1.16) | 1.81 (1.34) | p < 0.001 | NR |
| | | | Slowed Thinking/ Organization | 1.89 (1.18) | 1.11 (1.21) | p < 0.001 | NR |
| Nelson, Hoelzle, Doane, et al., 2012[29] | Axis I disorder | Memory | --- | 1 (5.6) | 4 (11.8) | "NS" | NR |
| Belanger, Proctor-Weber, Kretzmer, et al. 2011[12] | Blast exposure | NSI | Decision-Making | NR | NR | p > .002 | NR |
| | | | Memory | NR | NR | p > .002 | NR |
| | | | Slowed Thinking/ Organization | NR | NR | p > .002 | NR |
| Drag, Spencer, Walker, et al., 2012[20] | HADS Anxiety | NSI | Concentration | NR | NR | p < .001 | r = .56 |
| | | | Decision-Making | NR | NR | p < .001 | r = .52 |
| | | | Memory | NR | NR | p < .001 | r = .49 |
| | | | Slowed Thinking/ Organization | NR | NR | p < .001 | r = .58 |
| | HADS Depression | NSI | Concentration | NR | NR | p < .001 | r = .55 |
| | | | Decision-Making | NR | NR | p < .001 | r = .57 |
| | | | Memory | NR | NR | p < .001 | r = .51 |
| | | | Slowed Thinking/ Organization | NR | NR | p < .001 | r = .62 |
| | LOC and/or PTA | NSI | Concentration | 2.08 (1.21) | 2.71 (1.12) | NR | NR |
| | | | Decision-Making | 1.59 (1.365) | 2.05 (1.36) | NR | NR |
| | | | Memory | 2.17 (1.16) | 2.86 (1.18) | NR | NR |
| | | | Slowed Thinking/ Organization | 1.80 (1.32) | 2.38 (1.29) | NR | NR |
| Benge, Pastorek, & Thornton, 2009[13] | NA | NSI | Concentration | 2.31 (1.08) | NA | NA | NA |
| | | | Decision-Making | 1.72 (1.12) | NA | NA | NA |
| | | | Memory | 2.50 (1.04) | NA | NA | NA |
| | | | Slowed Thinking/ Organization | 1.96 (1.18) | NA | NA | NA |

| Author, year | Comparison group description | Outcome measure | Subscale or test component | mTBI group Mean (SD) | Comparison group Mean (SD) | p value for comparison | Magnitude of effect |
|---|---|---|---|---|---|---|---|
| Belanger, Proctor-Weber, Kretzmer, et al. 2011[12] | PCL score > 50 | NSI | Decision-Making | NR | NR | p < .002 | NR |
| | | | Memory | NR | NR | p < .002 | NR |
| | | | Slowed Thinking/ Organization | NR | NR | p < .002 | NR |
| Cooper, Kennedy, Cullen, et al., 2011[17] | PCL-C ≥60 (controls had PCL-C ≤30) | NSI | Cognitive Cluster | 3.04 (3.40) | 13.32 (3.90) | p < .0001 | NR |
| | | | Concentration | 0.47 (0.79) | 2.87 (0.88) | p < .0001 | NR |
| | | | Decision-Making | 0.33 (0.73) | 2.28 (1.13) | p < .0001 | NR |
| | | | Memory | 0.95 (1.14) | 3.00 (0.91) | p < .0001 | NR |
| | | | Slowed Thinking/ Organization | 0.42 (0.81) | 2.57 (0.98) | p < .0001 | NR |
| Drag, Spencer, Walker, et al., 2012[20] | PCL-M score | NSI | Concentration | NR | NR | p < .001 | r = .59 |
| | | | Decision-Making | NR | NR | p < .001 | r = .63 |
| | | | Memory | NR | NR | p < .001 | r = .53 |
| | | | Slowed Thinking/ Organization | NR | NR | p < .001 | r = .68 |
| Schiehser, Delis, Filoteo, et al., 2011[35] | Same population with moderate/severe TBI | FrSBe | Subjective Executive Dysfunction pre- to post-injury change | 10.8 (14.2) | 21.6 (18.3) | p = .01 | NR |
| Drag, Spencer, Walker, et al., 2012[20] | Service connected | NSI | Concentration | NR | NR | p < .05 | NR |
| | | | Decision-Making | NR | NR | p < .05 | NR |
| | | | Memory | NR | NR | p < .001 | NR |
| | | | Slowed Thinking/ Organization | NR | NR | p < .05 | NR |

## Physical Health Outcomes

Table 2a. Headache outcomes in studies of U.S. Veterans and members of the U.S. military with mild TBI

| Author, year | Comparison group description | Outcome measure | mTBI group Mean (SD) or % of subjects | Comparison group Mean (SD) or % of subjects | p value for comparison | Magnitude of effect |
|---|---|---|---|---|---|---|
| Kennedy, Cullen, Amador, et al., 2010[25] | At least one additional AIS code | NSI: Headaches | 2.71 (1.10) | 1.45 (1.30) | p < 0.001 | NR |
| Nelson, Hoelzle, Doane, et al., 2012[29] | Axis I disorder | Headache | 6 (33.3) | 12 (35.3) | "NS" | NR |
| Belanger, Proctor-Weber, Kretzmer, et al. 2011[12] | Blast exposure | NSI: Headaches | NR | NR | p < .002 | NR |
| Cooper, Chau, Armistead-Jehle, et al., 2012[16] | Blast exposure | HIT-6 | 54.32 (9.44) | 56.03 (9.54) | p = 0.489 | NR |
| Ruff, Ruff, & Wang, 2009[34] | Headache intervention involving sleep hygiene, Prazosin, headache and pain education, and group therapy | Headache frequency (number per month) | 12.40 (.94) | 4.77 (.19) | p < .001 | NR |
| | | Headache pain level (scale 0-10) | 7.28 (.27) | 4.08 (.19) | p < .001 | NR |
| Benge, Pastorek, & Thornton, 2009[13] | NA | NSI: Headaches | 2.29 (1.04) | NA | NA | NA |
| Patil, St. Andre, Crisen, et al., 2011[31] | NA | Neurology referral for headaches | 82/246 = 33.3% | NA | NA | NA |
| | | Neurology referral for headaches, Chronic daily type | 11/246 = 4.47% | NA | NA | NA |
| | | Neurology referral for headaches, Cluster type | 1/246 = 0.41% | NA | NA | NA |
| | | Neurology referral for headaches, Migraine type | 25/246 = 10.16% | NA | NA | NA |
| | | Neurology referral for headaches, Mixed type | 8/246 = 3.25% | NA | NA | NA |
| | | Neurology referral for headaches, Other type | 1/246 = 0.41% | NA | NA | NA |
| | | Neurology referral for headaches, Post-traumatic type | 4/246 = 1.63% | NA | NA | NA |
| | | Neurology referral for headaches, Tension type | 6/246 = 2.44% | NA | NA | NA |
| Theeler & Erickson, 2009[38] | NA | Headaches started < 1 week after trauma | 12/33 = 36% | NA | NA | NA |
| | | Headaches started > 1 month after trauma | 3/33 = 9% | NA | NA | NA |
| | | Headaches started 1 week to 1 month after trauma | 1/33 = 3% | NA | NA | NA |
| | | Unspecified onset of headache after trauma | 5/33 = 15% | NA | NA | NA |
| | | Worsening of pre-existing headaches | 12/33 = 36% | NA | NA | NA |
| Belanger, Proctor-Weber, Kretzmer et al. 2011[12] | PCL score > 50 | NSI: Headaches | NR | NR | p < .002 | NR |
| Cooper, Kennedy, Cullen, et al., 2011[17] | PCL-C ≥60 (controls had PCL-C ≤30) | NSI: Headaches | 1.01 (1.15) | 2.79 (1.18) | p < .0001 | NR |

# Complications of Mild Traumatic Brain Injury in Veterans and Military Personnel: A Systematic Review

| Author, year | Comparison group description | Outcome measure | mTBI group Mean (SD) or % of subjects | Comparison group Mean (SD) or % of subjects | p value for comparison | Magnitude of effect |
|---|---|---|---|---|---|---|
| Ruff, Ruff, & Wang, 2008[33] | Positive neurological and/or neuropsychological findings | Headache frequency: > 10 per month | 0/0 = 0% | 31/74 = 42% | p < .001 | NR |
| | | Headache frequency: > 4 per month | 2/6 = 33% | 71/74 = 96% | p < .001 | NR |
| | | Headache frequency: Daily | 0/0 = 0% | 10/14 = 14% | p < .001 | NR |
| | | Headache pain level (scale 0-10) | 4.33 (.27) | 7.28 (.27) | p < .001 | NR |
| | | Headache: Migraine type | 0/0 = 0% | 14/74 = 19% | p < .001 | NR |
| | | Headache: Mixed type | 0/0 = 0% | 30/74 = 41% | p < .001 | NR |
| | | Headache: Tension type | 6/6 = 100% | 30/74 = 41% | p < .001 | NR |
| Patil, St. Andre, Crisen, et al., 2011[31] | Referral to Neurology clinic for headaches | NSI: Headache | 1.97 (0.91) | 2.87 (0.80) | p < .01 | NR |
| Theeler & Erickson, 2009[38] | Same population without mTBI | Headache days per month after deployment (days/month) | 11.9 (10.0) | 10.3 (8.0) | NR | NR |
| | | Headache days per month during deployment (days/month) | 14.5 (11.7) | 9.4 (9.4) | NR | NR |
| | | Headache duration (hours) | 8.8 (7.3) | 7.5 (5.2) | NR | NR |
| | | Headache NOS | 7/33 = 21% | 7/48 = 14% | NR | NR |
| | | Headache severity (0-10 scale) | 7.1 (1.5) | 7.1 (1.2) | NR | NR |
| | | Medication overuse headache | 4/33 = 12% | 0/48 = 0% | NR | NR |
| | | MIDAS | 30.8 (44.3) | 26.8 (27.5) | NR | NR |
| | | Migraine with aura | 8/33 = 24% | 3/48 = 6% | NR | NR |
| | | Migraine without aura | 15/33 = 45% | 30/48 = 62% | NR | NR |
| | | Multiple headache types | 10/33 = 30% | 16/48 = 33% | NR | NR |
| | | Occipital headache | 5/33 = 15% | 3/48 = 6% | NR | NR |
| | | Probable migraine | 3/33 = 9% | 5/48 = 10% | NR | NR |
| | | Tension-type headache | 5/33 = 15% | 13/48 = 27% | NR | NR |

## Table 2b. Pain outcomes in studies of U.S. Veterans and members of the U.S. military with mild TBI

| Author, year | Comparison group description | Outcome measure | mTBI group | Comparison group | p value for comparison | Magnitude of effect |
|---|---|---|---|---|---|---|
| Barnes, Walter, & Chard, 2012[9] | Same population without mTBI | Pain (On a scale of 0 to 10, with 0 as no pain and 10 as the worst pain possible, how would you rate your current pain?) | Median = 3.5 | Median = 2.0 | p = .18 | Cohen's d = .30 |
| Lew, Pogoda, Hsu, et al., 2010[27] | Same population with moderate/severe TBI | Pain in the past 30-days | 112/125 = 90% | 6/6 = 100% | p = .53 | NR |

## Table 2c. Vestibular outcomes in studies of U.S. Veterans and members of the U.S. military with mild TBI

| Author, year | Comparison group description | Outcome measure | mTBI group Mean (SD) | Comparison group Mean (SD) | p value for comparison | Magnitude of effect |
|---|---|---|---|---|---|---|
| Belanger, Proctor-Weber, Kretzmer, et al. 2011[12] | Blast exposure | NSI: Feeling Dizzy | NR | NR | p > .002 | NR |
| | | NSI: Loss of Balance | NR | NR | p > .002 | NR |
| | | NSI: Poor Coordination | NR | NR | p > .002 | NR |
| | PCL score > 50 | NSI: Feeling Dizzy | NR | NR | p < .002 | NR |
| | | NSI: Loss of Balance | NR | NR | p < .002 | NR |
| | | NSI: Poor Coordination | NR | NR | p < .002 | NR |
| Benge, Pastorek, & Thornton, 2009[13] | NA | NSI: Feeling Dizzy | 1.47 (.86) | NA | NA | NA |
| | | NSI: Loss of Balance | 1.32 (.92) | NA | NA | NA |
| | | NSI: Poor Coordination | 1.32 (.93) | NA | NA | NA |
| Cooper, Kennedy, Cullen, et al., 2011[17] | PCL-C ≥60 (controls had PCL-C ≤30) | NSI: Feeling Dizzy | 0.52 (0.81) | 1.88 (1.13) | p < .0001 | NR |
| | | NSI: Loss of Balance | 0.45 (0.66) | 1.89 (1.04) | p < .0001 | NR |
| | | NSI: Poor Coordination | 0.30 (0.55) | 1.98 (1.04) | p < .0001 | NR |
| Gottshall, Drake, Gray, et al., 2003[23] | Control volunteer subjects without TBI. Not explicitly stated whether controls came from the same population as cases, but the controls were evaluated at the same time and place. | DHI | NR | NR | p < .01 for weeks 1, 2, 3, & 4 following injury | NR |
| | Control volunteer subjects without TBI. Not explicitly stated whether controls came from the same population as cases, but the controls were evaluated at the same time and place. | DVAT | NR | NR | p < .01 for week 1 / p > .01 for week 4 | NR |
| Kennedy, Cullen, Amador, et al., 2010[25] | At least one additional AIS code | NSI: Feeling Dizzy | 1.44 (1.09) | 0.94 (1.05) | p < 0.001 | NR |
| | | NSI: Loss of Balance | 1.30 (1.08) | 0.92 (0.98) | p = 0.002 | NR |
| | | NSI: Poor Coordination | 1.71 (1.05) | 0.92 (1.03) | p < 0.001 | NR |
| Nelson, Hoelzle, Doane, et al., 2012[29] | Axis I disorder | Disorientation | 7 (38.9) | 13 (38.2) | "NS" | NR |
| | | Dizziness | 5 (27.8) | 8 (23.5) | "NS" | NR |
| | | Imbalance | 2 (11.1) | 4 (11.8) | "NS" | NR |

## Table 2d. Vision outcomes in studies of U.S. Veterans and members of the U.S. military with mild TBI

| Author, year | Comparison group description | Outcome measure | mTBI group | Comparison group | p value for comparison | Magnitude of effect |
|---|---|---|---|---|---|---|
| Kennedy, Cullen, Amador, et al., 2010[25] | At least one additional AIS code | NSI: Sensitivity to Light | 1.56 (1.26) | 0.85 (1.22) | p < 0.001 | NR |
| | | NSI: Vision Problems | 1.18 (1.16) | 0.86 (1.16) | p = 0.022 | NR |
| Nelson, Hoelzle, Doane, et al., 2012[29] | Axis I disorder | Photophobia | 4 (22.2) | 6 (17.6) | "NS" | NR |
| Belanger, Proctor-Weber, Kretzmer, et al. 2011[12] | Blast exposure | NSI: Sensitivity to Light | NR | NR | p > .002 | NR |
| | | NSI: Vision Problems | NR | NR | p > .002 | NR |
| Benge, Pastorek, & Thornton, 2009[13] | NA | NSI: Sensitivity to Light | 1.72 (1.17) | NA | NA | NA |
| | | NSI: Vision Problems | 1.51 (1.07) | NA | NA | NA |
| Belanger, Proctor-Weber, Kretzmer, et al., 2011[12] | PCL score > 50 | NSI: Sensitivity to Light | NR | NR | p < .002 | NR |
| | | NSI: Vision Problems | NR | NR | p < .002 | NR |
| Cooper, Kennedy, Cullen, et al., 2011[17] | PCL-C ≥60 (controls had PCL-C ≤30) | NSI: Sensitivity to Light | 0.65 (0.99) | 2.06 (1.44) | p < .0001 | NR |
| | | NSI: Vision Problems | 0.51 (0.99) | 1.68 (1.23) | p < .0001 | NR |

## Table 2e. Hearing outcomes in studies of U.S. Veterans and members of the U.S. military with mild TBI

| Author, year | Comparison group description | Outcome measure | | mTBI group Mean (SD) | Comparison group Mean (SD) | p value for comparison | Magnitude of effect |
|---|---|---|---|---|---|---|---|
| Belanger, Proctor-Weber, Kretzmer, et al., 2011[12] | Blast exposure | NSI | Hearing Difficulty | NR | NR | p < .002 | NR |
| | | | Sensitivity to Noise | NR | NR | p > .002 | NR |
| | PCL score > 50 | NSI | Hearing Difficulty | NR | NR | p < .002 | NR |
| | | | Sensitivity to Noise | NR | NR | p < .002 | NR |
| Benge, Pastorek, & Thornton, 2009[13] | NA | NSI | Hearing Difficulty | 1.88 (1.06) | NA | NA | NA |
| | | | Sensitivity to Noise | 1.85 (1.11) | NA | NA | NA |
| Cooper, Kennedy, Cullen, et al., 2011[17] | PCL-C ≥60 (controls had PCL-C ≤30) | NSI | Sensitivity to Noise | 0.48 (0.87) | 2.50 (1.09) | p < .0001 | NR |
| | | | Hearing Difficulty | 0.70 (1.02) | 2.06 (1.11) | p < .0001 | NR |
| Kennedy, Cullen, Amador, et al., 2010[25] | At least one additional AIS code | NSI | Sensitivity to Noise | 1.86 (1.17) | 1.29 (1.41) | p < 0.001 | NR |
| | | | Hearing Difficulty | 1.46 (1.12) | 1.39 (1.28) | p = 0.620 | NR |
| Nelson, Hoelzle, Doane, et al., 2012[29] | Axis I disorder | | Tinnitus | 8 (44.4) | 13 (38.2) | "NS" | NR |
| | | | Phonophobia | 4 (22.2) | 4 (11.8) | "NS" | NR |

## Table 2f. Neurological outcomes in studies of U.S. Veterans and members of the U.S. military with mild TBI

| Author, year | Comparison group description | Outcome measure | mTBI group Mean (SD) or % of subjects | Comparison group Mean (SD) or % of subjects | p value for comparison | Magnitude of effect |
|---|---|---|---|---|---|---|
| Kennedy, Cullen, Amador, et al., 2010[25] | At least one additional AIS code | NSI: Numbness or Tingling | 1.02 (1.08) | 1.22 (1.32) | p = 0.157 | NR |
| Belanger, Proctor-Weber, Kretzmer, et al., 2011[12] | Blast exposure | NSI: Numbness or Tingling | NR | NR | p > .002 | NR |
| Ruff, Riechers, Wang, et al., 2012[32] | LOC | Neurological deficits based on examination | 0/16 = 0% | 65/125 = 52% | p < .001 | NR |
| Benge, Pastorek, & Thornton, 2009[13] | NA | NSI: Numbness or Tingling | 1.61 (1.19) | NA | NA | NA |
| Belanger, Proctor-Weber, Kretzmer, et al., 2011[12] | PCL score > 50 | NSI: Numbness or Tingling | NR | NR | p < .002 | NR |
| Cooper, Kennedy, Cullen, et al., 2011[17] | PCL-C ≥60 (controls had PCL-C ≤30) | NSI: Numbness or Tingling | 0.76 (0.96) | 1.83 (1.26) | p < .0001 | NR |

## Table 2g. Nausea/appetite outcomes in studies of U.S. Veterans and members of the U.S. military with mild TBI

| Author, year | Comparison group description | | Outcome measure | mTBI group Mean (SD) | Comparison group Mean (SD) | p value for comparison | Magnitude of effect |
|---|---|---|---|---|---|---|---|
| Belanger, Proctor-Weber, Kretzmer, et al., 2011[12] | Blast exposure | NSI | Change in Taste or Smell | NR | NR | p > .002 | NR |
| | | | Loss of Appetite | NR | NR | p > .002 | NR |
| | | | Nausea | NR | NR | p > .002 | NR |
| | PCL score > 50 | NSI | Change in Taste or Smell | NR | NR | p < .002 | NR |
| | | | Loss of Appetite | NR | NR | p < .002 | NR |
| | | | Nausea | NR | NR | p < .002 | NR |
| Benge, Pastorek, & Thornton, 2009[13] | NA | NSI | Change in Taste or Smell | 0.82 (1.03) | NA | NA | NA |
| | | | Loss of Appetite | 1.53 (1.13) | NA | NA | NA |
| | | | Nausea | 1.13 (1.01) | NA | NA | NA |
| Cooper, Kennedy, Cullen, et al., 2011[17] | PCL-C ≥60 (controls had PCL-C ≤30) | NSI | Change in Taste or Smell | 0.15 (0.60) | 1.14 (1.14) | p < .0001 | NR |
| | | | Loss of Appetite | 0.50 (0.84) | 2.05 (1.10) | p < .0001 | NR |
| | | | Nausea | 0.31 (0.70) | 1.57 (1.12) | p < .0001 | NR |
| Kennedy, Cullen, Amador, et al., 2010[25] | At least one additional AIS code | NSI | Change in Taste or Smell | 0.54 (0.92) | 0.49 (0.90) | p = 0.681 | NR |
| | | | Loss of Appetite | 1.44 (1.11) | 1.13 (1.16) | p = 0.026 | NR |
| | | | Nausea | 1.12 (1.07) | 0.60 (0.94) | p < 0.001 | NR |
| Nelson, Hoelzle, Doane, et al., 2012[29] | Axis I disorder | | Nausea | 3 (16.7) | 4 (11.8) | "NS" | NR |

## Mental Health Outcomes

**Table 3a. PTSD outcomes in studies of U.S. Veterans and members of the U.S. military with mild TBI**

| Author, year | Comparison group description | | Outcome measure | mTBI group Mean (SD) | Comparison group Mean (SD) | p value for comparison | Magnitude of effect |
|---|---|---|---|---|---|---|---|
| Kennedy, Cullen, Amador, et al., 2010[25] | At least one additional AIS code | PCL-C | Arousal With Reminder | 3.02 (1.39) | 2.17 (1.36) | p < 0.001 | NR |
| | | | Avoid Activities | 2.50 (1.39) | 2.03 (1.28) | p = 0.004 | NR |
| | | | Avoid Thoughts | 2.92 (1.42) | 2.31 (1.36) | p < 0.001 | NR |
| | | | Avoidance Cluster | 17.72 (7.54) | 13.93 (6.61) | p < 0.001 | NR |
| | | | Disturbing Dreams | 3.10 (1.42) | 2.74 (1.47) | p = 0.042 | NR |
| | | | Disturbing Memories | 3.32 (1.32) | 3.03 (1.43) | p = 0.086 | NR |
| | | | Feeling Distant | 2.97 (1.43) | 2.10 (1.22) | p < 0.001 | NR |
| | | | Feeling Numb | 2.31 (1.41) | 1.85 (1.19) | p = 0.004 | NR |
| | | | Future Cut Short | 2.29 (1.40) | 1.85 (1.24) | p = 0.006 | NR |
| | | | Hyper-Arousal Cluster | 17.47 (4.91) | 13.65 (5.58) | p < 0.001 | NR |
| | | | Irritability | 3.18 (1.32) | 2.51 (1.40) | p < 0.001 | NR |
| | | | Jumpy, Easily Startled | 3.34 (1.30) | 2.72 (1.41) | p < 0.001 | NR |
| | | | Loss of Interest | 2.55 (1.41) | 2.01 (1.19) | p = 0.001 | NR |
| | | | Poor Sleep | 4.11 (1.16) | 3.36 (1.48) | p < 0.001 | NR |
| | | | Re-experiencing Cluster | 14.95 (5.74) | 12.07 (5.92) | p < 0.001 | NR |
| | | | Reliving Experience | 2.54 (1.29) | 1.99 (1.26) | p < 0.001 | NR |
| | | | Super-Alert, Watchful | 3.44 (1.28) | 2.67 (1.39) | p < 0.001 | NR |
| | | | Total Score | 50.14 (16.66) | 39.64 (16.72) | p < 0.001 | NR |
| | | | Trouble Concentrating | 3.41 (1.26) | 2.46 (1.39) | p < 0.001 | NR |
| | | | Trouble Remembering | 2.48 (1.42) | 2.05 (1.32) | p = 0.009 | NR |
| | | | Upset When Reminded | 2.98 (1.34) | 2.42 (1.36) | p = 0.001 | NR |
| Nelson, Hoelzle, Doane, et al., 2012[29] | Axis I disorder | | CAPS | 9.8 (12.1) | 54.2 (52.5) | "Significant" | NR |
| | | | SCID-I: PTSD | 0 (0.0) | 24 (70.6) | "NS" | NR |
| Belanger, Proctor-Weber, Kretzmer, et al., 2011[12] | Blast exposure | | PCL | 37.3 (17.6) | 41.5 (17.4) | p = .047 | NR |
| Cooper, Chau, Armistead-Jehle, et al., 2012[16] | Blast exposure | | PCL-M | 36.29 (14.72) | 37.88 (16.42) | p = .696 | NR |

# Complications of Mild Traumatic Brain Injury in Veterans and Military Personnel: A Systematic Review

Evidence-based Synthesis Program

| Author, year | Comparison group description | Outcome measure | | mTBI group Mean (SD) | Comparison group Mean (SD) | p value for comparison | Magnitude of effect |
|---|---|---|---|---|---|---|---|
| Kennedy, Leal, Lewis, et al., 2010[26] | Blast exposure | PCL-C | Avoidance | All: 15.6 (7.0) AOC: 14.8 (6.9) LOC: 16.1 (7.1) | All: 15.8 (7.4) AOC: 14.9 (7.1) LOC: 16.3 (7.5) | All: p = .826 AOC: "NS" LOC: "NS" | NR |
| | | | Hyper-Arousal | All: 14.5 (5.7) AOC: 14.0 (5.6) LOC: 14.8 (5.8) | All: 15.2 (5.6) AOC: 14.6 (5.4) LOC: 15.6 (5.7) | All: p = .202 AOC: "NS" LOC: "NS" | NR |
| | | | Re-experiencing | All: 12.0 (5.7) AOC: 11.8 (5.8) LOC: 12.2 (5.8) | All: 13.3 (5.9) AOC: 12.6 (5.7) LOC: 13.7 (5.9) | All: p = .020 AOC: "NS" LOC: "NS" | NR |
| | | | Total Score | All: 42.7 (16.9) AOC: 40.6 (17.0) LOC: 43.1 (17.0) | All: 44.3 (17.6) AOC: 42.0 (16.8) LOC: 45.7 (17.9) | All: p = .198 AOC: "NS" LOC: "NS" | NR |
| Lippa, Pasternik, Benge, & Thornton, 2010[28] | Blast exposure | PCL: Civilian and Military versions | | 49.75 (15.11) | 54.45 (14.98) | p = .005 | NR |
| Drag, Spencer, Walker, et al., 2012[20] | HADS Anxiety | PCL-M | | NR | NR | p < .001 | r = .76 |
| | HADS Depression | PCL-M | | NR | NR | p < .001 | r = .76 |
| Ruff, Riechers, Wang, et al., 2012[32] | LOC | PTSD diagnosis (based on PCL-M as well as clinical interview) | | 1/16 = 6.25% | 83/125 = 66% | p < .001 | NR |
| Drag, Spencer, Walker, et al., 2012[20] | LOC and/or PTA | PCL-M | | 50.61 (16.24) | 56.74 (14.61) | p < .05 | NR |
| Benge, Pastorek, & Thornton, 2009[13] | NA | PCL-C: Total Score | | 53.5 (15.6) | NA | NA | NA |
| Spencer et al., 2010[36] | NA | PCL-M | | 52.4 (15.0) | NA | NA | NA |
| Ruff, Ruff, & Wang, 2008[33] | Positive neurological and/or neuropsychological findings | PTSD diagnosis: (PCL score > 50 and meeting DSM-IV criteria) | | 11/46 = 24% | 72/80 = 90% | p < .001 | NR |
| Patil, St. Andre, Crisen, et al., 2011[31] | Referral to neurology clinic for headaches | PTSD (clinician confirmed or self-reported symptoms) | | 116/164 = 70.7% | 66/82 = 80.5% | p = .10 | NR |
| Belanger, Kretzmer, Venderploeg, & French, 2010[10] | Same population with moderate/severe TBI | PCL | | 35.4 (16.8) | 23.5 (13.7) | p < .0001 | NR |
| Belanger, Kretzmer, Yoash-Gantz, Pickett, & Tupler, 2009[11] | Same population with moderate/severe TBI | PCL | | 45.5 (17.2) | 30.1 (15.5) | p < .0001 | NR |
| Cooper, Nelson, Armistead-Jehle, & Bowles, 2011[19] | Same population with moderate/severe TBI | PCL-M | | 42 (1) | 37 (3) | NR | NR |
| Lew, Pogoda Hsu, et al., 2010[27] | Same population with moderate/severe TBI | PTSD diagnosis | | 91/125 = 73% | 5/6 = 83% | p = .49 | NR |
| Cooper, Nelson, Armistead-Jehle, & Bowles, 2011[19] | Same population without mTBI | PCL-M | | 42 (1) | 31 (4) | NR | NR |
| Gaylord, 2008[21] | Same population without mTBI | PCL-M: Score </= 44 | | 14/31 = 45% | 10/45 = 22% | p = .0345 | NR |
| Theeler & Erickson, 2009[38] | Same population without mTBI | PCL-C | | 34.6 (13.3) | 36.0 (14.0) | NR | NR |

| Author, year | Comparison group description | Outcome measure | mTBI group Mean (SD) | Comparison group Mean (SD) | p value for comparison | Magnitude of effect |
|---|---|---|---|---|---|---|
| Barnes, Walter, & Chard, 2012[9] | Same population without mTBI | CAPS: B – Re-experiencing Subscale | 20.02 (7.03) | 17.53 (6.06) | p = .08 | Cohen's d = 0.38 |
| | | CAPS: Total Score | 74.02 (16.21) | 67.20 (13.21) | p = .03 | Cohen's d = 0.46 |
| | | PCL-S | 61.86 (11.04) | 58.19 (12.89) | p = .17 | Cohen's d = 0.30 |
| Cooper, Nelson, Armistead-Jehle, & Bowles, 2011[19] | Same population, neurologic patients (tumor, stroke, electrical, subarachnoid hemorrhage, anoxia, encephalitis, Parkinson's disease, fronto-temporal dementia) | PCL-M | 42 (1) | 35 (5) | NR | NR |
| Spencer et al., 2010[36] | Self-reported attention deficits | PCL-M | NR | NR | p < .001 | r = .60 |
| | Self-reported memory deficits | PCL-M | NR | NR | p < .001 | r = .48 |
| | Self-reported slowed thinking/ organization | PCL-M | NR | NR | p < .001 | r = .54 |

## Table 3b. Measures of anxiety in studies of U.S. Veterans and members of the U.S. military with mild TBI

| Author, year | Comparison group description | Outcome measure | mTBI group Mean (SD) | Comparison group Mean (SD) | p value for comparison | Magnitude of effect |
|---|---|---|---|---|---|---|
| Belanger, Proctor-Weber, Kretzmer, et al., 2011[12] | Blast exposure | NSI: Feeling Anxious | NR | NR | "NS" | NR |
| | PCL score > 50 | NSI: Feeling Anxious | NR | NR | p < .002 | NR |
| Benge, Pastorek, & Thornton, 2009[13] | NA | NSI: Feeling Anxious | 2.58 (1.08) | NA | NA | NA |
| Cooper, Kennedy, Cullen, et al., 2011[17] | PCL-C ≥60 (controls had PCL-C ≤30) | NSI: Feeling Anxious | 0.48 (0.82) | 2.96 (0.91) | p < .0001 | NR |
| Drag, Spencer, Walker, et al., 2012[20] | LOC and/or PTA | HADS: Anxiety | 11.56 (4.06) | 13.16 (3.92) | p < .05 | NR |
| | HADS Depression | HADS: Anxiety | NR | NR | p < .001 | r = .56 |
| Kennedy, Cullen, Amador, et al., 2010[25] | At least one additional AIS code | NSI: Feeling Anxious | 1.99 (1.24) | 1.49 (1.34) | p = 0.001 | NR |
| Spencer, et al., 2010[36] | NA | HADS: Anxiety | 11.9 (4.5) | NA | NA | NA |
| | Self-reported slowed thinking/organization | HADS: Anxiety | NR | NR | p < .001 | r = .39 |
| | Self-reported attention deficits | HADS: Anxiety | NR | NR | p < .001 | r = .48 |
| | Self-reported memory deficits | HADS: Anxiety | NR | NR | p < .001 | r = .33 |

## Table 3c. Measures of depression in studies of U.S. Veterans and members of the U.S. military with mild TBI

| Author, year | Comparison group description | Outcome measure | Subscale or test component | mTBI group Mean (SD) or % of subjects | Comparison group Mean (SD) or % of subjects | p value for comparison | Magnitude of effect |
|---|---|---|---|---|---|---|---|
| Kennedy, Cullen, Amador, et al., 2010[25] | At least one additional AIS code | NSI | Feeling Depressed or Sad | 1.16 (1.26) | 1.08 (1.19) | p = 0.566 | NR |
| Belanger, Proctor-Weber, Kretzmer, et al., 2011[12] | Blast exposure | NSI | Feeling Depressed or Sad | NR | NR | "NS" | NR |
| Drag, Spencer, Walker, et al., 2012[20] | LOC and/or PTA | HADS | Depression | 7.95 (4.61) | 10.34 (4.013) | p < .001 | NR |
| Benge, Pastorek, & Thornton, 2009[13] | NA | NSI | Feeling Depressed or Sad | 2.09 (1.20) | NA | NA | NA |
| Spencer et al., 2010[36] | NA | HADS | Depression | 8.7 (4.3) | NA | NA | NA |
| Belanger, Proctor-Weber, Kretzmer, et al., 2011[12] | PCL score > 50 | NSI | Feeling Depressed or Sad | NR | NR | p < .002 | NR |
| Cooper, Kennedy, Cullen, et al., 2011[17] | PCL-C ≥60 (controls had PCL-C ≤30) | NSI | Depression | 0.30 (0.64) | 2.44 (1.19) | p < .0001 | NR |
| Swick, Honzel, Larsen, et al., 2012[37] | Same population without mTBI; all participants had PTSD. | BDI-II | --- | 20.0 (12.3) | 20.8 (9.2) | NR | NR |
| Barnes, Walter, & Chard, 2012[9] | Same population without mTBI | BDI-II | --- | 31.56 (11.06) | 29.17 (10.53) | p = .29 | Cohen's d = 0.23 |
| | | Hopelessness (Who or what gives you strength and hope?) | --- | 6/46 = 13% | 6/46 = 13% | NR | NR |
| | | SCID-I | Major Depressive Disorder | 25/46 = 54% | 18/46 = 39% | p = .14 | φ = .15 |
| Spencer, et al., 2010[36] | Self-reported attention deficits | HADS | Depression | NR | NR | p < .001 | r = .45 |
| | Self-reported memory deficits | HADS | Depression | NR | NR | p < .001 | r = .36 |
| | Self-reported slowed thinking/organization | HADS | Depression | NR | NR | p < .001 | r = .52 |

## Table 3d. Substance use disorders in studies of U.S. Veterans and members of the U.S. military with mild TBI

| Author, year | Comparison group description | Outcome measure | Subscale or test component | mTBI group % of subjects | Comparison group % of subjects | p value for comparison | Magnitude of effect |
|---|---|---|---|---|---|---|---|
| Nelson, Hoelzle, Doane, et al., 2012[29] | Axis I disorder | SCID-I | Alcohol Abuse/Dependence | 5/18 = 27.8% | 12/34 = 35.3% | "Significant" | NR |
| | Same population without mTBI; none have Axis I | | Alcohol Abuse/Dependence | 5/18 = 27.8% | 5/28 = 17.9% | "NS" | NR |
| Barnes, Walter, & Chard, 2012[9] | Same population without mTBI | SCID-I | Alcohol Problem | 13/46 = 28% | 17/46 = 37% | p = .37 | φ = .09 |
| | | | Drug Problem | 4/46 = 9% | 7/46 = 15% | p = .34 | φ = .10 |

## Table 3e. Suicide-related outcomes in studies of U.S. Veterans and members of the U.S. military with mild TBI

| Author, year | Comparison group description | Outcome measure | mTBI group % of subjects | Comparison group % of subjects | p value for comparison | Magnitude of effect |
|---|---|---|---|---|---|---|
| Barnes, Walter, & Chard, 2012[9] | Same population without mTBI | Suicidal ideation (Have you had thoughts about death or about killing yourself?) | 11/44 = 25% | 5/44 = 11% | p = .10 | φ = .18 |
| | | Suicidal Intent (Have you ever intended to commit suicide?) | 3/46 = 7% | 1/46 = 2% | NR | NR |
| | | Past Suicide Attempts (Have you ever attempted suicide?) | 2/46 = 4% | 2/46 = 4% | NR | NR |

## Table 3f. Other mental health outcomes in studies of U.S. Veterans and members of the U.S. military with mild TBI

| Author, year | Comparison group description | Outcome measure | Subscale or test component | mTBI group | Comparison group | p value for comparison | Magnitude of effect |
|---|---|---|---|---|---|---|---|
| Kennedy, Cullen, Amador, et al., 2010[25] | At least one additional AIS code | NSI | Affective Cluster | 7.21 (4.21) | 5.43 (4.54) | p < 0.001 | NR |
| | | | Frustration | 1.86 (1.22) | 1.24 (1.29) | p < 0.001 | NR |
| | | | Irritability | 2.19 (1.23) | 1.62 (1.32) | p < 0.001 | NR |
| Belanger, Proctor-Weber, Kretzmer, et al. 2011[12] | Blast exposure | NSI | Frustration | NR | NR | "NS" | NR |
| Benge, Pastorek, & Thornton, 2009[13] | NA | NSI | Frustration | 2.41 (1.17) | NA | NA | NA |
| | | | Irritability | 2.76 (1.06) | NA | NA | NA |
| Belanger, Proctor-Weber, Kretzmer, et al. 2011[12] | PCL score > 50 | NSI | Frustration | NR | NR | p < .002 | NR |
| Cooper, Kennedy, Cullen, et al., 2011[17] | PCL-C ≥60 (controls had PCL-C ≤30) | NSI | Affective Cluster | 2.97 (2.93) | 14.64 (3.48) | p < .0001 | NR |
| | | | Frustration | 0.31 (0.68) | 2.82 (0.95) | p < .0001 | NR |
| | | | Irritability | 0.63 (0.89) | 2.95 (0.90) | p < .0001 | NR |
| Schiehser, Delis, Filoteo, et al., 2011[35] | Same population with moderate/severe TBI | FrSBe | Apathy, pre- to post-injury change | 14.7 (17.2) | 27.8 (16.8) | p < .01 | NR |
| | | | Behavioral Disinhibition, pre- to post-injury change | 5.3 (7.8) | 5.5 (11.2) | p = .98 | NR |
| Barnes, Walter, & Chard, 2012[9] | Same population without mTBI | SCID-I | Any Co-Morbid Axis I Disorder | 34/46 = 78% | 29/46 = 63% | p = .14 | φ = .12 |
| Cooper, Mercado-Couch, Critchfield, et al., 2010[18] | Same population without mTBI | Psychiatric Diagnosis | --- | 25 (50.0%) | 26 (22.2%) | p = 0.001 | NR |

## Functional/Social Outcomes

**Table 4a. Employment outcomes in studies of U.S. Veterans and members of the U.S. military with mild TBI**

| Author, year | Comparison group description | Outcome measure | mTBI group % of subjects or OR (95% CI) compared to non-mTBI control | Comparison group % of subjects or OR (95% CI) compared to non-mTBI control | p value for comparison | Magnitude of effect |
|---|---|---|---|---|---|---|
| Barnes, Walter, & Chard, 2012[9] | Same population without mTBI | Unemployment (% who responded 'No' to 'Are you employed?') | 9/45 = 20% | 14/45 = 31% | p = .23 | φ = .13 |
| Toblin, Riviere, Thomas, et al., 2012[39] | LOC | Missed work: ≥2 missed workdays in the past month | 1.8 (95% CI 0.9-3.5) | 1.4 (95% CI 0.5-3.6) | NR | NR |
| | | Occupational Impairment, Heavy Load: Difficulty carrying a heavy load in past month | 2.2 (95% CI 1.3-3.5) | 3.0 (95% CI 1.5-5.7) | NR | NR |
| | | Occupational Impairment, Physical Training: Difficulty performing physical training (PT) in past month | 1.9 (95% CI 1.2-2.9) | 1.6 (95% CI 0.8-3.0) | NR | NR |

104

**Table 4b. Sleep outcomes in studies of U.S. Veterans and members of the U.S. military with mild TBI**

| Author, year | Comparison group description | Outcome measure | Subscale or test component | mTBI group Mean (SD), Median (IQR), or % of subjects | Comparison group Mean (SD), Median (IQR), or % of subjects | p value for comparison | Magnitude of effect |
|---|---|---|---|---|---|---|---|
| Kennedy, Cullen, Amador, et al., 2010[25] | At least one additional AIS code | NSI | Fatigue | 1.85 (1.11) | 1.51 (1.14) | p = 0.009 | NR |
| | | | Sleep | 2.73 (1.10) | 2.15 (1.33) | p < 0.001 | NR |
| Belanger, Proctor-Weber, Kretzmer, et al. 2011[12] | Blast exposure | NSI | Fatigue | NR | NR | p < .002 | NR |
| Ruff, Ruff, & Wang, 2009[34] | Headache intervention involving sleep hygiene, Prazosin, headache and pain education, and group therapy | ESS | --- | 16.10 (0.28) | 7.28 (0.34) | p < .001 | NR |
| Benge, Pastorek, & Thornton, 2009[13] | NA | NSI | Fatigue | 2.10 (1.11) | NA | NA | NA |
| | | | Sleep | 2.72 (1.17) | NA | NA | NA |
| Coldren, Russell, Parish, et al., 2012[15] | Same population without mTBI; with minor traumatic injuries not involving the head and noninjured volunteers from same population | Sleep | hours per night < 4 | 6/47 = 13% | 7/108 = 7% | p = 0.21 for sleep hours overall | NR |
| | | | hours per night ≥4 | 40/47 = 87% | 99/108 = 93% | p = 0.21 for sleep hours overall | NR |
| | | Sleep Change | < 2 hour loss | 10/47 = 23% | 4/108 = 6% | p = 0.02 for sleep change overall | NR |
| | | | > 2 hour loss | 33/47 = 77% | 62/108 = 94% | p = 0.02 for sleep change overall | NR |
| Kelly, Coldren, Parish, et al., 2012[24] | Same population without mTBI; with minor traumatic injuries not involving the head and noninjured volunteers from same population | Sleep | hours per night | Median = 6 (5-7) | Median = 6 (5-7) | p = .22 | NR |
| | | Sleep Change (negative value = hours lost) | --- | Median = 0 (-2.5-0) | Median = 0 (0-0) | p < 0.001 | NR |
| Belanger, Proctor-Weber, Kretzmer, et al., 2011[12] | PCL score > 50 | NSI | Fatigue | NR | NR | p < .002 | NR |
| Cooper, Kennedy, Cullen, et al., 2011[17] | PCL-C ≥60 (controls had PCL-C ≤30) | NSI | Fatigue | 0.86 (0.91) | 2.60 (1.04) | p < .0001 | NR |
| | | | Sleep | 1.24 (1.17) | 3.45 (0.70) | p < .0001 | NR |
| Ruff, Ruff, & Wang, 2008[33] | Positive neurological and/or neuropsychological findings | NSI | Sleep | 5/46 = 11% | 66/80 = 82.5% | p < .001 | NR |
| Patil, St. Andre, Crisen, et al., 2011[31] | Referral to Neurology clinic for headaches | NSI | Sleep | 2.53 (1.17) | 2.78 (1.12) | p = .11 | NR |
| Lew, Pogoda Hsu, et al., 2010[27] | Same population with moderate/severe TBI | Sleep disturbance in the past 30 days | --- | 2.72 (1.24) | 3.17 (.75) | p = .38 | NR |

### Table 4c. Social outcomes in studies of U.S. Veterans and members of the U.S. military with mild TBI

| Author, year | Comparison group description | Outcome measure | mTBI group % of subjects | Comparison group % of subjects | p value for comparison | Magnitude of effect |
|---|---|---|---|---|---|---|
| Barnes, Walter, & Chard, 2012[9] | Same population without mTBI | Lack of emotional support (% who responded 'No' to 'Do you have an emotional support system?') | 9/35 = 26% | 6/35 = 17% | p = .38 | φ = .10 |
| | | Marital status (Are you married?) | NR | NR | p = .72 | φ = .04 |

## Service Utilization/Costs

### Table 5. Service utilization outcomes in studies of U.S. Veterans and members of the U.S. military with mild TBI

| Author, year | Comparison group description | Outcome Measure | mTBI group OR (95% CI) compared to non-mTBI control, % of subjects, or Mean (SD) | Comparison group OR (95% CI) compared to non-mTBI control, % of subjects, or Mean (SD) | p value for comparison | Magnitude of effect |
|---|---|---|---|---|---|---|
| Toblin, Riviere, Thomas, et al., 2012[39] | LOC | Medical utilization: ≥2 "sick call" visits in past month | 2.0 (95% CI 1.3-3.1) | 1.9 (95% CI 1.04-3.6) | NR | NR |
| Coldren, Russell, Parish, et al., 2012[15] | Same population without mTBI; with minor traumatic injuries not involving the head and noninjured volunteers from same population | Current Counseling | 2/47 = 4% | 4/108 = 4% | p >0.99 | NR |
| | | Current Mental Health Medication | 2/47 = 4% | 9/108 = 9% | p = 0.50 | NR |
| Kelly, Coldren, Parish, et al., 2012[24] | Same population without mTBI; with minor traumatic injuries not involving the head and noninjured volunteers from same population | Current Counseling | 4/66 = 6% | 5/146 = 3% | p = .46 | NR |
| | | Current Mental Health Medication | 3/66 = 5% | 8/146 = 6% | p = .99 | NR |
| Belanger, Kretzmer, Venderploeg, & French, 2010[10] | Same population with moderate/severe TBI | Currently taking pain medications | 24/44 = 55% | 37/64 = 57% | p = .44 | NR |
| Gaylord 2008[21] | Same population without mTBI | Length of Hospital Stay (days) | PTSD: 13.6 (9.8) No PTSD: 19.0 (20.9) | PTSD: 16.0 (26.6) No PTSD: 14.1 (22.2) | NR | NR |
| | | Length of Intensive Care Unit Stay (days) | PTSD: 2.0 (6.7) No PTSD: 12.1 (12.1) | PTSD: 1.6 (3.9) No PTSD: 2.8 (8.9) | NR | NR |
| Swick, Honzel, Larsen, et al., 2012[37] | Same population without mTBI; all participants had PTSD. | Number of medications | 18 | 5 | NR | NR |
| Cooper, Mercado-Couch, Critchfield, et al., 2010[18] | Same population without mTBI | Pain Medication (Narcotic) | 32 (64.0%) | 85 (72.6%) | p = 0.264 | NR |

# APPENDIX F. LIST OF EXCLUDED STUDIES GROUPED BY REASON FOR EXCLUSION

| *Population does not meet criteria for adult, human subjects who are Veterans or members of the military from any country* |
| --- |
| Axelrod BN, Vanderploeg RD, Rawlings DB. WAIS-R prediction equations in patients with traumatic brain injury. *J Clin Exp Neuropsychol.* Jun 1999;21(3):368-374. |
| Belanger HG, Curtiss G, Demery JA, Lebowitz BK, Vanderploeg RD. Factors moderating neuropsychological outcomes following mild traumatic brain injury: a meta-analysis. *J Int Neuropsychol Soc.* May 2005;11(3):215-227. |
| Belanger HG, Spiegel E, Vanderploeg RD. Neuropsychological performance following a history of multiple self-reported concussions: a meta-analysis. *J Int Neuropsychol Soc.* Mar 2010;16(2):262-267. |
| Binder LM. Assessment of malingering after mild head trauma with the Portland Digit Recognition Test.[Erratum appears in J Clin Exp Neuropsychol 1993 Nov;15(6):852]. *J Clin Exp Neuropsychol.* Mar 1993;15(2):170-182. |
| Bryan C, Anestis M. Reexperiencing symptoms and the interpersonal-psychological theory of suicidal behavior among deployed service members evaluated for traumatic brain injury. *J Clin Psychol.* Sep 2011;67(9):856-865. |
| Bryan C, Hernandez AM. Magnitudes of decline on Automated Neuropsychological Assessment Metrics subtest scores relative to predeployment baseline performance among service members evaluated for traumatic brain injury in Iraq. *J Head Trauma Rehabil.* Jan-Feb 2012;27(1):45-54. |
| Bryan CJ, Clemans TA, Hernandez AM. Perceived burdensomeness, fearlessness of death, and suicidality among deployed military personnel. *Personality and Individual Differences.* Feb 2012;52(3):374-379. |
| Bryan CJ, Hernandez AM. Predictors of post-traumatic headache severity among deployed military personnel. *Headache.* Jun 2011;51(6):945-953. |
| Cho DY, Wang YC. Comparison of the APACHE III, APACHE II and Glasgow Coma Scale in acute head injury for prediction of mortality and functional outcome. *Intensive Care Med.* Jan 1997;23(1):77-84. |
| Crawford F, Crynen G, Reed J, et al. Identification of plasma biomarkers of TBI outcome using proteomic approaches in an APOE mouse model. *J Neurotrauma.* Jan 20 2012;29(2):246-260. |
| Dobscha SK, Clark ME, Morasco BJ, Freeman M, Campbell R, Helfand M. Systematic review of the literature on pain in patients with polytrauma including traumatic brain injury. *Pain Med.* Oct 2009;10(7):1200-1217. |
| Eagleman DM. Using time perception to measure fitness for duty. *Military Psychology.* Jan 2009;21(Suppl 1):S123-S129. |
| Gervasio AH, Kreutzer JS. Kinship and family members' psychological distress after traumatic brain injury: A large sample study. *The Journal of Head Trauma Rehabilitation.* Jun 1997;12(3):14-26. |
| Hoffer ME, Gottshall KR, Moore R, Balough BJ, Wester D. Characterizing and treating dizziness after mild head trauma. *Otol Neurotol.* Mar 2004;25(2):135-138. |
| Hoffman JM, Lucas S, Dikmen S, et al. Natural history of headache after traumatic brain injury. *J Neurotrauma.* Sep 2011;28(9):1719-1725. |
| Kane RL, Roebuck-Spencer T, Short P, Kabat M, Wilken J. Identifying and monitoring cognitive deficits in clinical populations using Automated Neuropsychological Assessment Metrics (ANAM) tests. *Arch Clin Neuropsychol.* Feb 2007;22 Suppl 1:S115-126. |

Kreutzer JS, Marwitz JH, Hsu N, Williams K, Riddick A. Marital stability after brain injury: an investigation and analysis. *NeuroRehabilitation.* 2007;22(1):53-59.

Lew HL, Chen CPC, Chen MJL, Hsu THC, Tang SFT, Date ES. Comparing the effects of different speech targets on cognitive event-related potentials: theoretical implications for evaluating brain injury. *Am J Phys Med Rehabil.* Jul 2002;81(7):524-528.

Lew HL, Gray M, Poole JH. Temporal stability of auditory event-related potentials in healthy individuals and patients with traumatic brain injury. *J Clin Neurophysiol.* Oct 2007;24(5):392-397.

Lew HL, Thomander D, Gray M, Poole JH. The effects of increasing stimulus complexity in event-related potentials and reaction time testing: clinical applications in evaluating patients with traumatic brain injury. *J Clin Neurophysiol.* Oct 2007;24(5):398-404.

Lewine JD, Davis JT, Bigler ED, et al. Objective documentation of traumatic brain injury subsequent to mild head trauma: multimodal brain imaging with MEG, SPECT, and MRI. *J Head Trauma Rehabil.* May-Jun 2007;22(3):141-155.

Luethcke CA, Bryan CJ, Morrow CE, Isler WC. Comparison of Concussive Symptoms, Cognitive Performance, and Psychological Symptoms Between Acute Blast-Versus Nonblast-Induced Mild Traumatic Brain Injury. *J Int Neuropsychol Soc.* 2011;17(1):36-45.

Maas AI, Harrison-Felix CL, Menon D, et al. Common data elements for traumatic brain injury: recommendations from the interagency working group on demographics and clinical assessment. *Arch Phys Med Rehabil.* Nov 2010;91(11):1641-1649.

Montella D, Brown SH, Elkin PL, et al. Comparison of SNOMED CT versus Medcin terminology concept coverage for mild Traumatic Brain Injury. *AMIA Annu Symp Proc.* 2011;2011:969-978.

Norman SB, Trim RS, Goldsmith AA, et al. Role of risk factors proximate to time of trauma in the course of PTSD and MDD symptoms following traumatic injury. *J Trauma Stress.* Aug 2011;24(4):390-398.

Schmid KE, Tortella FC. The diagnosis of traumatic brain injury on the battlefield. *Front Neurol.* 2012;3:90.

Smith-Seemiller L, Fow NR, Kant R, Franzen MD. Presence of post-concussion syndrome symptoms in patients with chronic pain vs mild traumatic brain injury. *Brain Inj.* 2003;17(3):199-206.

*Publication contains no primary data and is not a systematic review of primary studies*

Aksionoff EB, Falk NS. The differential diagnosis of perceptual deficits in traumatic brain injury patients. *J Am Optom Assoc.* Aug 1992;63(8):554-558.

Anonymous. Cognitive rehabilitation therapy in traumatic brain injury. *The Lancet.* Oct 2011;378(9801):1440.

Anonymous. The neurological burden of the war in Iraq and Afghanistan. *Ann Neurol.* Oct 2006;60(4):A13-15.

Arcure J, Harrison EE. A review of the use of early hypothermia in the treatment of traumatic brain injuries. *J Spec Oper Med.* 2009;9(3):22-25.

Barr M. Post concussion syndrome hypoglycemia and Agent Orange. *Aust Fam Physician.* Apr 1983;12(4):224.

Barrett RS. Post-traumatic headache. Combat soldiers are suffering. *Adv NPs PAs.* Jan 2012;3(1):33-34.

Belanger HG, Uomoto JM, Vanderploeg RD. The Veterans Health Administration's (VHA's) Polytrauma System of Care for mild traumatic brain injury: costs, benefits, and controversies. *J Head Trauma Rehabil.* Jan-Feb 2009;24(1):4-13.

Belanger HG, Vanderploeg RD, Curtiss G, Warden DL. Recent neuroimaging techniques in mild traumatic brain injury. *J Neuropsychiatry Clin Neurosci.* 2007;19(1):5-20.

Betthauser LM, Bahraini N, Krengel MH, Brenner LA. Self-report measures to identify post traumatic stress disorder and/or mild traumatic brain injury and associated symptoms in military veterans of Operation Enduring Freedom (OEF)/Operation Iraqi Freedom (OIF). *Neuropsychol Rev.* Mar 2012;22(1):35-53.

Bhattacharjee Y. Neuroscience. Shell shock revisited: solving the puzzle of blast trauma. *Science.* Jan 25 2008;319(5862):406-408.

Bogdanova Y, Verfaellie M. Cognitive sequelae of blast-induced traumatic brain injury: recovery and rehabilitation. *Neuropsychol Rev.* Mar 2012;22(1):4-20.

Brancu M, Straits-Troster K, Kudler H. Behavioral health conditions among military personnel and veterans: prevalence and best practices for treatment. *N C Med J.* Jan-Feb 2011;72(1):54-60.

Brenner LA, Vanderploeg RD, Terrio H. Assessment and diagnosis of mild traumatic brain injury, posttraumatic stress disorder, and other polytrauma conditions: burden of adversity hypothesis. *Rehabil Psychol.* Aug 2009;54(3):239-246.

Brenner LA. Neuropsychological and neuroimaging findings in traumatic brain injury and post-traumatic stress disorder. *Dialogues Clin Neurosci.* 2011;13(3):311-323.

Bryant RA. Disentangling mild traumatic brain injury and stress reactions. *The New England Journal of Medicine.* Jan 2008;358(5):525-527.

Caldroney RD, Radike J. Experience with mild traumatic brain injuries and postconcussion syndrome at Kandahar, Afghanistan. *US Army Med Dep J.* Jul-Sep 2010:22-30.

Cancio LC, Chung KK. The role of normoventilation in improving traumatic brain injury outcomes. *US Army Med Dep J.* Apr-Jun 2011:49-54.

Cernich AN, Kurtz SM, Mordecai KL, Ryan PB. Cognitive rehabilitation in traumatic brain injury. *Curr Treat Options Neurol.* Sep 2010;12(5):412-423.

Cifu DX, Cohen SI, Lew HL, Jaffee M, Sigford B. The history and evolution of traumatic brain injury rehabilitation in military service members and veterans. *Am J Phys Med Rehabil.* Aug 2010;89(8):688-694.

Connors S, Gordon WA, Hovda DA. Care of war veterans with mild traumatic brain injury. *N Engl J Med.* Jul 30 2009;361(5):536-537; author reply 537-538.

Cooke BB, Keltner NL. Biological perspectives: traumatic brain injury-war related: part II. *Perspect Psychiatr Care.* Jan 2008;44(1):54-57.

Cote MJ, Syam SS, Vogel WB, Cowper DC. A mixed integer programming model to locate traumatic brain injury treatment units in the Department of Veterans Affairs: a case study. *Health Care Manag Sci.* Sep 2007;10(3):253-267.

Cozzarelli TA. Evaluation and treatment of persistent cognitive dysfunction following mild traumatic brain injury. *J Spec Oper Med.* 2010;10(1):39-42.

Daggett V, Bakas T, Habermann B. A review of health-related quality of life in adult traumatic brain injury survivors in the context of combat veterans. *J Neurosci Nurs.* Apr 2009;41(2):59-71.

Das RR. Mild traumatic brain injury in U.S. soldiers returning from Iraq. *N Engl J Med.* May 15 2008;358(20):2177-2178; author reply 2179.

Dempsey KE, Dorlac WC, Martin K, et al. Landstuhl Regional Medical Center: traumatic brain injury screening program. *J Trauma Nurs.* Jan-Mar 2009;16(1):6-7, 10-12.

Department of Veterans A. Schedule for rating disabilities; evaluation of residuals of traumatic brain injury (TBI). Final rule. *Fed Regist.* Sep 23 2008;73(185):54693-54708.

Dolan S, Martindale S, Robinson J, et al. Neuropsychological sequelae of PTSD and TBI following war deployment among OEF/OIF veterans. *Neuropsychol Rev.* Mar 2012;22(1):21-34.

Doster J. Traumatic brain injury: serving our returning soldiers. *Tenn Med.* Oct 2007;100(10):45, 48.

Eibner C, Schell TL, Jaycox LH. Care of war veterans with mild traumatic brain injury. *N Engl J Med.* Jul 30 2009;361(5):537; author reply 537-538.

Eldar R, Jelic M. The association of rehabilitation and war. *Disabil Rehabil.* Sep 16 2003;25(18):1019-1023.

Evans RW. Posttraumatic headaches among United States soldiers injured in Afghanistan and Iraq. *Headache: The Journal of Head and Face Pain.* Sep 2008;48(8):1216-1225.

Felber ES. Combat-related posttraumatic headache: diagnosis, mechanisms of injury, and challenges to treatment. *J Am Osteopath Assoc.* Dec 2010;110(12):737-738.

Giles GM. Cognitive versus functional approaches to rehabilitation after traumatic brain injury: Commentary on a randomized controlled trial. *Am J Occup Ther.* Jan-Feb 2010;64(1):182-185.

Graham DP, Cardon AL. An update on substance use and treatment following traumatic brain injury. *Ann N Y Acad Sci.* Oct 2008;1141:148-162.

Graver CJ. "Reference data from the Automated Neuropsychological Assessment Metrics for use in traumatic brain injury in an active duty military sample": Comment. *Mil Med.* Dec 2009;174(12):iv-v.

Helmick K, Members of Consensus C. Cognitive rehabilitation for military personnel with mild traumatic brain injury and chronic post-concussional disorder: Results of April 2009 consensus conference. *NeuroRehabilitation.* 2010;26(3):239-255.

Hesdorffer DC, Rauch SL, Tamminga CA. Long-term psychiatric outcomes following traumatic brain injury: a review of the literature. *J Head Trauma Rehabil.* Nov-Dec 2009;24(6):452-459.

Hicks RR, Fertig SJ, Desrocher RE, Koroshetz WJ, Pancrazio JJ. Neurological effects of blast injury. *J Trauma.* May 2010;68(5):1257-1263.

Hoge CW, Castro CA. Blast-related traumatic brain injury in U.S. military personnel. *N Engl J Med.* Sep 1 2011;365(9):860; author reply 860-861.

Hoge CW, Goldberg HM, Castro CA. Care of war veterans with mild traumatic brain injury--flawed perspectives. *N Engl J Med.* Apr 16 2009;360(16):1588-1591.

Hoge CW. "Traumatic brain injury screening: Preliminary findings in a US Army Brigade Combat Team": Comment. *The Journal of Head Trauma Rehabilitation.* Jul-Aug 2009;24(4):299-301.

Jackson GL, Hamilton NS, Tupler LA. Detecting traumatic brain injury among veterans of Operations Enduring and Iraqi Freedom. *N C Med J.* Jan-Feb 2008;69(1):43-47.

Jaffee MS, Helmick KM, Girard PD, Meyer KS, Dinegar K, George K. Acute clinical care and care coordination for traumatic brain injury within Department of Defense. *J Rehabil Res Dev.* 2009;46(6):655-666.

Jasiewicz J, Kearns W, Craighead J, Fozard JL, Scott S, McCarthy J, Jr. Smart rehabilitation for the 21st century: the Tampa Smart Home for veterans with traumatic brain injury. *J Rehabil Res Dev.* 2011;48(8):vii-xviii.

Kaplan GB, Vasterling JJ, Vedak PC. Brain-derived neurotrophic factor in traumatic brain injury, post-traumatic stress disorder, and their comorbid conditions: role in pathogenesis and treatment. *Behav Pharmacol.* Sep 2010;21(5-6):427-437.

Kelly JC, Amerson EH, Barth JT. Mild traumatic brain injury: lessons learned from clinical, sports, and combat concussions. *rehabil.* 2012;2012:371970.

Kirjavainen S. Neuro-otological studies on brain injured ex-servicemen. Follow-up of 256 cases. *Acta Otolaryngol (Stockh).* 1968:Suppl 233:231-259.

Krainin BM, Forsten RD, Kotwal RS, Lutz RH, Guskiewicz KM. Mild traumatic brain injury literature review and proposed changes to classification. *J Spec Oper Med.* 2011;11(3):38-47.

Leung LY, VandeVord PJ, Dal Cengio AL, Bir C, Yang KH, King AI. Blast related neurotrauma: a review of cellular injury. *Mol Cell Biomech.* Sep 2008;5(3):155-168.

Lew HL, Vanderploeg RD, Moore DF, et al. Overlap of mild TBI and mental health conditions in returning OIF/OEF service members and veterans. *J Rehabil Res Dev.* 2008;45(3):xi-xvi.

Lew HL, Weihing J, Myerse PJ, Pogoda TK, Goodrich GL. Dual sensory impairment (DSI) in traumatic brain injury (TBI)-An emerging interdisciplinary challenge. *NeuroRehabilitation.* 2010;26(3):213-222.

Lew HL. Rehabilitation needs of an increasing population of patients: Traumatic brain injury, polytrauma, and blast-related injuries. *J Rehabil Res Dev.* Jul-Aug 2005;42(4):xiii-xvi.

Lutz RH, Kane S, Lay J. Evidence-based diagnosis and management of mTBI in forward deployed settings: the genesis of the USASOC neurocognitive testing and post-injury evaluation and treatment program. *J Spec Oper Med.* 2010;10(1):23-38.

McCrea M, Pliskin N, Barth J, et al. Official position of the military TBI task force on the role of neuropsychology and rehabilitation psychology in the evaluation, management, and research of military veterans with traumatic brain injury. *Clin Neuropsychol.* Jan 2008;22(1):10-26.

Miller G. Neuropathology. Blast injuries linked to neurodegeneration in veterans. *Science.* May 18 2012;336(6083):790-791.

Miller G. The invisible wounds of war. Healing the brain, healing the mind. *Science.* Jul 29 2011;333(6042):514-517.

Okie S. Traumatic brain injury in the war zone. *N Engl J Med.* May 19 2005;352(20):2043-2047.

Pogoda TK, Vanderploeg RD, Cifu DX, Tun CG, Lew HL. Re: separating deployment-related traumatic brain injury and posttraumatic stress disorder in veterans: preliminary findings from the VA TBI screening program. *Am J Phys Med Rehabil.* Dec 2009;88(12):1043-1044; author reply 1044-1045.

Robinson RG, Jorge R. Longitudinal course of mood disorders following traumatic brain injury. *Arch Gen Psychiatry.* Jan 2002;59(1):23-24.

Ropper A. Brain injuries from blasts. *N Engl J Med.* Jun 2 2011;364(22):2156-2157.

Ruff RL. Mild traumatic brain injury in U.S. soldiers returning from Iraq. *N Engl J Med.* May 15 2008;358(20):2178; author reply 2179.

Ruff RM, Iverson GL, Barth JT, Bush SS, Broshek DK. Recommendations for diagnosing a mild traumatic brain injury: A National Academy of Neuropsychology education paper. *Arch Clin Neuropsychol.* Feb 2009;24(1):3-10.

Sayer NA, Rettmann NA, Carlson KF, et al. Veterans with history of mild traumatic brain injury and posttraumatic stress disorder: challenges from provider perspective. *J Rehabil Res Dev.* 2009;46(6):703-716.

Shenton M, Hamoda H, Schneiderman J, et al. A review of magnetic resonance imaging and diffusion tensor imaging findings in mild traumatic brain injury. *Brain Imaging and Behavior.* Jun 2012;6(2):137-192.

Sigford B, Cifu DX, Vanderploeg R. Care of war veterans with mild traumatic brain injury. *N Engl J Med.* Jul 30 2009;361(5):536; author reply 537-538.

SoRelle R. Head injuries linked to Alzheimer's disease. *Circulation.* Oct 31 2000;102(18):E9036-9037.

Stelmack J. Measuring outcomes of neuro-optometric care in traumatic brain injury. *Journal of Behavioral Optometry.* 2007;18(3):67-71.

Stonesifer LD. Mild traumatic brain injury in U.S. soldiers returning from Iraq. *N Engl J Med.* May 15 2008;358(20):2178; author reply 2179.

Taber KH, Hurley RA. PTSD and combat-related injuries: functional neuroanatomy. *J Neuropsychiatry Clin Neurosci.* 2009;21(1):1 p preceding 1, 1-4.

Walcott BP, Kahle KT. Blast-related traumatic brain injury in U.S. military personnel. *N Engl J Med.* Sep 1 2011;365(9):860.

Walker RL, Clark ME, Nampiaparampil DE, et al. The hazards of war: blast injury headache. *J Pain.* Apr 2010;11(4):297-302.

Xydakis MS, Butman JA, Carlo P. Blast-related traumatic brain injury in U.S. military personnel. *The New England Journal of Medicine.* Sep 2011;365(9):859.

### *Does not distinguish mild TBI from moderate or severe*

Alterman AI, Tarter RE. Relationship between familial alcoholism and head injury. *Journal of Studies on Alcohol.* May 1985;46(3):256-258.

Armistead-Jehle P, Hansen CL. Comparison of the Repeatable Battery for the Assessment of Neuropsychological Status Effort Index and stand-alone symptom validity tests in a military sample. *Arch Clin Neuropsychol.* Nov 2011;26(7):592-601.

Ashla PM, McMurtray AM, Licht E, Mendez MF. Retrospective posttraumatic amnesia in traumatic brain injury. *The Journal of Neuropsychiatry and Clinical Neurosciences.* Fal 2009;21(4):467-468.

Belanger HG, King-Kallimanis B, Nelson AL, Schonfeld L, Scott SG, Vanderploeg RD. Characterizing wandering behaviors in persons with traumatic brain injury residing in veterans health administration nursing homes. *Arch Phys Med Rehabil.* Feb 2008;89(2):244-250.

Belanger HG, Vanderploeg RD, Soble JR, Richardson M, Groer S. Validity of the Veterans Health Administration's traumatic brain injury screen. *Arch Phys Med Rehabil.* Jul 2012;93(7):1234-1239.

Blennow K, Jonsson M, Andreasen N, et al. No neurochemical evidence of brain injury after blast overpressure by repeated explosions or firing heavy weapons. *Acta Neurol Scand.* Apr 2011;123(4):245-251.

Braden CA, Cuthbert JP, Brenner L, et al. Health and wellness characteristics of persons with traumatic brain injury. *Brain Inj.* 2012;26(11):1315-1327.

Brahm KD, Wilgenburg HM, Kirby J, Ingalla S, Chang C-Y, Goodrich GL. Visual impairment and dysfunction in combat-injured servicemembers with traumatic brain injury. *Optom Vis Sci.* Jul 2009;86(7):817-825.

Brenner LA, Betthauser LM, Homaifar BY, et al. Posttraumatic stress disorder, traumatic brain injury, and suicide attempt history among veterans receiving mental health services. *Suicide Life Threat Behav.* Aug 2011;41(4):416-423.

Brenner LA, Homaifar BY, Adler LE, Wolfman JH, Kemp J. Suicidality and veterans with a history of traumatic brain injury: precipitants events, protective factors, and prevention strategies. *Rehabil Psychol.* Nov 2009;54(4):390-397.

Brenner LA, Ignacio RV, Blow FC. Suicide and traumatic brain injury among individuals seeking Veterans Health Administration services. *J Head Trauma Rehabil.* Jul-Aug 2011;26(4):257-264.

Breshears RE, Brenner LA, Harwood JEF, Gutierrez PM. Predicting suicidal behavior in veterans with traumatic brain injury: the utility of the personality assessment inventory. *J Pers Assess.* Jul 2010;92(4):349-355.

Brooks E. Understanding veterans' service options and utilization patterns for PTSD and TBI. *Dissertation Abstracts International: Section B: The Sciences and Engineering.* 2011;71(8-B):4739.

Campbell TA, Nelson LA, Lumpkin R, Yoash-Gantz RE, Pickett TC, McCormick CL. Neuropsychological measures of processing speed and executive functioning in combat veterans with PTSD, TBI, and comorbid TBI/PTSD. *Psychiatric Annals.* Aug 2009;39(8):796-803.

Capaldi VF, 2nd, Guerrero ML, Killgore WDS. Sleep disruptions among returning combat veterans from Iraq and Afghanistan. *Mil Med.* Aug 2011;176(8):879-888.

Carey ME, Young HF, Mathis JL. The outcome of 89 American and 224 Vietnamese sustaining brain wounds in Vietnam. *Mil Med.* Apr 1974;139(4):281-284.

Carey ME, Young HF, Rish BL, Mathis JL. Follow-up study of 103 American soldiers who sustained a brain wound in Vietnam. *J Neurosurg.* Nov 1974;41(5):542-549.

Carlson KF, Meis LA, Jensen AC, et al. Caregiver reports of subsequent injuries among veterans with traumatic brain injury after discharge from inpatient polytrauma rehabilitation programs. *J Head Trauma Rehabil.* Jan-Feb 2012;27(1):14-25.

Carlson KF, Nelson D, Orazem RJ, Nugent S, Cifu DX, Sayer NA. Psychiatric diagnoses among Iraq and Afghanistan war veterans screened for deployment-related traumatic brain injury. *J Trauma Stress.* Feb 2010;23(1):17-24.

Caveness WF, Walker AE, Ascroft PB. Incidence of posttraumatic epilepsy in Korean veterans as compared with those from World War I and World War II. *J Neurosurg.* Feb 1962;19:122-129.

Cernich AN, Chandler L, Scherdell T, Kurtz S. Assessment of co-occurring disorders in veterans diagnosed with traumatic brain injury. *J Head Trauma Rehabil.* Jul-Aug 2012;27(4):253-260.

Chauhan NB, Gatto R. Synergistic benefits of erythropoietin and simvastatin after traumatic brain injury. *Brain Res.* Nov 11 2010;1360:177-192.

Chemtob CM, Muraoka MY, Wu-Holt P, Fairbank JA, Hamada RS, Keane TM. Head injury and combat-related posttraumatic stress disorder. *J Nerv Ment Dis.* Nov 1998;186(11):701-708.

Chen JWY, Ruff RL, Eavey R, Wasterlain CG. Posttraumatic epilepsy and treatment. *J Rehabil Res Dev.* 2009;46(6):685-696.

Cohen SP, Plunkett AR, Wilkinson I, et al. Headaches during war: analysis of presentation, treatment, and factors associated with outcome. *Cephalalgia.* Jan 2012;32(2):94-108.

Cox DJ, Davis M, Singh H, et al. Driving rehabilitation for military personnel recovering from traumatic brain injury using virtual reality driving simulation: a feasibility study. *Mil Med.* Jun 2010;175(6):411-416.

Crawford FC, Vanderploeg RD, Freeman MJ, et al. APOE genotype influences acquisition and recall following traumatic brain injury. *Neurology.* Apr 9 2002;58(7):1115-1118.

Cullen N, Chundamala J, Bayley M, Jutai J, Erabi G. The efficacy of acquired brain injury rehabilitation. *Brain Inj.* Feb 2007;21(2):113-132.

Das RR, Moorthi RN. Traumatic brain injury in the war zone. *N Engl J Med.* Aug 11 2005;353(6):633-634.

Demakis GJ, Hammond F, Knotts A, et al. The Personality Assessment Inventory in individuals with traumatic brain injury. *Arch Clin Neuropsychol.* Jan 2007;22(1):123-130.

Detweiler MB, Arif S, Candelario J, et al. Salem VAMC-U.S. Army Fort Bragg Warrior Transition Clinic telepsychiatry collaboration: 12-month operation clinical perspective. *Telemed J E Health.* Mar 2012;18(2):81-86.

Donnelly KT, Donnelly JP, Dunnam M, et al. Reliability, sensitivity, and specificity of the VA traumatic brain injury screening tool. *J Head Trauma Rehabil.* Nov-Dec 2011;26(6):439-453.

Drake AI, Meyer KS, Cessante LM, et al. Routine TBI screening following combat deployments. *NeuroRehabilitation.* 2010;26(3):183-189.

Egede LE, Dismuke C, Echols C. Racial/Ethnic disparities in mortality risk among US veterans with traumatic brain injury. *Am J Public Health.* May 2012;102 Suppl 2:S266-271.

Elbogen EB, Johnson SC, Wagner HR, Newton VM, Beckham JC. Financial well-being and postdeployment adjustment among Iraq and Afghanistan war veterans. *Mil Med.* Jun 2012;177(6):669-675.

Elbogen EB, Wagner HR, Fuller SR, et al. Correlates of anger and hostility in Iraq and Afghanistan war veterans. *Am J Psychiatry.* Sep 2010;167(9):1051-1058.

Eonta SE, Carr W, McArdle JJ, et al. Automated Neuropsychological Assessment Metrics: repeated assessment with two military samples. *Aviat Space Environ Med.* Jan 2011;82(1):34-39.

Ettinger AB, Copeland LA, Zeber JE, Van Cott AC, Pugh MJV. Are psychiatric disorders independent risk factors for new-onset epilepsy in older individuals? *Epilepsy Behav.* Jan 2010;17(1):70-74.

Evans CD. Rehabilitation of the brain-damaged survivor. *Injury.* Nov 1976;8(2):80-97.

Fabing HD. Cerebral blast syndrome in combat soldiers. *Arch Neurol Psychiatry.* Jan 1947;57(1):14-57.

Fenimore EA. Depression following traumatic brain injury and the Hamilton Depression Rating Scale. *Dissertation Abstracts International: Section B: The Sciences and Engineering.* 2006;67(3-B):1698.

Friedemann-Sanchez G, Sayer NA, Pickett T. Provider perspectives on rehabilitation of patients with polytrauma. *Arch Phys Med Rehabil.* Jan 2008;89(1):171-178.

Galarneau MR, Woodruff SI, Dye JL, Mohrle CR, Wade AL. Traumatic brain injury during Operation Iraqi Freedom: findings from the United States Navy-Marine Corps Combat Trauma Registry. *J Neurosurg.* May 2008;108(5):950-957.

Gallaway MS, Fink DS, Millikan AM, Bell MR. Factors Associated With Physical Aggression Among US Army Soldiers. *Aggress Behav.* Sep 2012;38(5):357-367.

Goldstein G, Allen DN, Caponigro JM. A retrospective study of heterogeneity in neurocognitive profiles associated with traumatic brain injury. *Brain Inj.* 2010;24(4):625-635.

Gontkovsky ST, Souheaver GT. T-score and raw-score comparisons in detecting brain dysfunction using the booklet category test and the short category test. *Percept Mot Skills.* Feb 2002;94(1):319-322.

Gordon NG. Diagnostic efficiency of the Trail Making Test as a function of cut-off score, diagnosis, and age. *Percept Mot Skills.* Aug 1978;47(1):191-195.

Griffin JM, Friedemann-Sanchez G, Jensen AC, et al. The invisible side of war: families caring for US service members with traumatic brain injuries and polytrauma. *J Head Trauma Rehabil.* Jan-Feb 2012;27(1):3-13.

Gutierrez PM, Brenner LA, Huggins JA. A preliminary investigation of suicidality in psychiatrically hospitalized veterans with traumatic brain injury. *Arch.* 2008;12(4):336-343.

Han SD, Suzuki H, Drake AI, Jak AJ, Houston WS, Bondi MW. Clinical, cognitive, and genetic predictors of change in job status following traumatic brain injury in a military population. *J Head Trauma Rehabil.* Jan-Feb 2009;24(1):57-64.

Harmon A. A descriptive study of military family needs following a polytraumatic injury. *Dissertation Abstracts International: Section B: The Sciences and Engineering.* 2008;69(2-B):1326.

Harrow JJ, Rashka SL, Fitzgerald SG, Nelson AL. Pressure ulcers and occipital alopecia in Operation Iraqi Freedom polytrauma casualties. *Mil Med.* Nov 2008;173(11):1068-1072.

Hill JJ, 3rd, Mobo BHP, Jr., Cullen MR. Separating deployment-related traumatic brain injury and posttraumatic stress disorder in veterans: preliminary findings from the Veterans Affairs traumatic brain injury screening program. *Am J Phys Med Rehabil.* Aug 2009;88(8):605-614.

Holsinger T, Steffens DC, Phillips C, et al. Head injury in early adulthood and the lifetime risk of depression. *Arch Gen Psychiatry.* Jan 2002;59(1):17-22.

Huckans M, Pavawalla S, Demadura T, et al. A pilot study examining effects of group-based Cognitive Strategy Training treatment on self-reported cognitive problems, psychiatric symptoms, functioning, and compensatory strategy use in OIF/OEF combat veterans with persistent mild cognitive disorder and history of traumatic brain injury. *J Rehabil Res Dev.* 2010;47(1):43-60.

Huggins JM, Brown JN, Capehart B, Townsend ML, Legge J, Melnyk SD. Medication adherence in combat veterans with traumatic brain injury. *Am J Health-Syst Pharm.* Feb 1 2011;68(3):254-258.

Ingala AM. The impact of military deployment on college adjustment. *Dissertation Abstracts International: Section B: The Sciences and Engineering.* 2012;72(11-B):7083.

Iverson KM, Hendricks AM, Kimerling R, et al. Psychiatric diagnoses and neurobehavioral symptom severity among OEF/OIF VA patients with deployment-related traumatic brain injury: a gender comparison. *Womens Health Issues.* Jul-Aug 2011;21(4 Suppl):S210-217.

Johns JS, Cifu DX, Keyser-Marcus L, Jolles PR, Fratkin MJ. Impact of clinically significant heterotopic ossification on functional outcome after traumatic brain injury. *J Head Trauma Rehabil.* Jun 1999;14(3):269-276.

Jones A, Ingram M, Ben-Porath YS. Scores on the MMPI-2-RF Scales as a function of increasing levels of failure on cognitive symptom validity tests in a military sample. *The Clinical Neuropsychologist.* Jul 2012;26(5):790-815.

Kalkonde YV, Jawaid A, Qureshi SU, et al. Medical and environmental risk factors associated with frontotemporal dementia: A case-control study in a veteran population. *Alzheimer's dement.* May 2012;8(3):204-210.

Kapidzic A, Vidovic M, Sinanovic O. Localisation of war craniocerebral injury as risk factor for posttraumatic epilepsy. *Med Arh.* 2011;65(6):343-344.

Kelley AM, Athy JR, Cho TH, Erickson B, King M, Cruz P. Risk propensity and health risk behaviors in U.S. army soldiers with and without psychological disturbances across the deployment cycle. *J Psychiatr Res.* May 2012;46(5):582-589.

Kennedy JE, Lumpkin RJ, Grissom JR. A survey of mild traumatic brain injury treatment in the emergency room and primary care medical clinics. *Mil Med.* Jun 2006;171(6):516-521.

Kilts JD, Tupler LA, Keefe FJ, et al. Neurosteroids and self-reported pain in veterans who served in the U.S. Military after September 11, 2001. *Pain Med.* Oct 2010;11(10):1469-1476.

King PR, Donnelly KT, Donnelly JP, et al. Psychometric study of the Neurobehavioral Symptom Inventory. *JRRD.* 2012;49(6):879-888.

King PR, Jr. A psychometric study of the Neurobehavioral Symptom Inventory. *Dissertation Abstracts International: Section B: The Sciences and Engineering.* 2012;73(1-B):650.

Koenigs M, Huey ED, Raymont V, et al. Focal brain damage protects against post-traumatic stress disorder in combat veterans. *Nat Neurosci.* Feb 2008;11(2):232-237.

Kozminski M. Combat-related posttraumatic headache: diagnosis, mechanisms of injury, and challenges to treatment. *J Am Osteopath Assoc.* Sep 2010;110(9):514-519.

Kraft JF, Schwab KA, Salazar AM, Brown HR. Occupational and educational achievements of head injured Vietnam veterans at 15-year follow-up. *Arch Phys Med Rehabil.* Jun 1993;74(6):596-601.

Levin HS, Wilde E, Troyanskaya M, et al. Diffusion tensor imaging of mild to moderate blast-related traumatic brain injury and its sequelae. *J Neurotrauma.* Apr 2010;27(4):683-694.

Lew HL, Jerger JF, Guillory SB, Henry JA. Auditory dysfunction in traumatic brain injury. *J Rehabil Res Dev.* 2007;44(7):921-928.

Lew HL, Kraft M, Pogoda TK, Amick MM, Woods P, Cifu DX. Prevalence and characteristics of driving difficulties in Operation Iraqi Freedom/Operation Enduring Freedom combat returnees. *J Rehabil Res Dev.* 2011;48(8):913-925.

Lew HL, Otis JD, Tun C, Kerns RD, Clark ME, Cifu DX. Prevalence of chronic pain, posttraumatic stress disorder, and persistent postconcussive symptoms in OIF/OEF veterans: polytrauma clinical triad. *J Rehabil Res Dev.* 2009;46(6):697-702.

Lew HL, Pogoda TK, Baker E, et al. Prevalence of dual sensory impairment and its association with traumatic brain injury and blast exposure in OEF/OIF veterans. *J Head Trauma Rehabil.* Nov-Dec 2011;26(6):489-496.

Lew HL, Poole JH, Vanderploeg RD, et al. Program development and defining characteristics of returning military in a VA Polytrauma Network Site. *J Rehabil Res Dev.* 2007;44(7):1027-1034.

Lipsky RH, Sparling MB, Ryan LM, et al. Association of COMT Val158Met genotype with executive functioning following traumatic brain injury. *J Neuropsychiatry Clin Neurosci.* 2005;17(4):465-471.

Maestas KL, Benge JF, Pastorek NJ, Lemaire A, Darrow R. Factor structure of posttraumatic stress disorder symptoms in OEF/OIF veterans presenting to a polytrauma clinic. *Rehabil Psychol.* Nov 2011;56(4):366-373.

Maguen S, Lau KM, Madden E, Seal K. Factors associated with completing comprehensive traumatic brain injury evaluation. *Mil Med.* Jul 2012;177(7):797-803.

Maguen S, Madden E, Lau KM, Seal K. The impact of head injury mechanism on mental health symptoms in veterans: do number and type of exposures matter? *J Trauma Stress.* Feb 2012;25(1):3-9.

Mantyla M. Post-traumatic cerebral atrophy. A study on brain-injured veterans on the Finnish wars of 1939-40 and 1941-45. *Ann Clin Res.* 1981;13(32):1-47.

Maxwell TM. The investigation of mild traumatic brain injury among the Afghanistan and Iraqi war veterans. *Dissertation Abstracts International: Section B: The Sciences and Engineering.* 2011;72(6-B):3778.

McMurtray A, Clark DG, Christine D, Mendez MF. Early-onset dementia: frequency and causes compared to late-onset dementia. *Dement Geriatr Cogn Disord.* 2006;21(2):59-64.

Meterko M, Baker E, Stolzmann KL, Hendricks AM, Cicerone KD, Lew HL. Psychometric assessment of the Neurobehavioral Symptom Inventory-22: the structure of persistent postconcussive symptoms following deployment-related mild traumatic brain injury among veterans. *J Head Trauma Rehabil.* Jan-Feb 2012;27(1):55-62.

Miller KJ, Schwab KA, Warden DL. Predictive value of an early Glasgow Outcome Scale score: 15-month score changes. *J Neurosurg.* Aug 2005;103(2):239-245.

Morissette SB, Woodward M, Kimbrel NA, et al. Deployment-related TBI, persistent postconcussive symptoms, PTSD, and depression in OEF/OIF veterans. *Rehabil Psychol.* Nov 2011;56(4):340-350.

Nelson DV, Esty ML. Neurotherapy of traumatic brain injury/posttraumatic stress symptoms in OEF/OIF veterans. *J Neuropsychiatry Clin Neurosci.* Mar 1 2012;24(2):237-240.

Nelson LA, Yoash-Gantz RE, Pickett TC, Campbell TA. Relationship between processing speed and executive functioning performance among OEF/OIF veterans: implications for postdeployment rehabilitation. *J Head Trauma Rehabil.* Jan-Feb 2009;24(1):32-40.

Nuutila A, Huusko S. Epilepsy among brain-injured veterans 26 to 31 years following the injury. *Scand J Rehabil Med.* 1972;4(2):81-84.

Olson-Madden JH, Brenner L, Harwood JEF, Emrick CD, Corrigan JD, Thompson C. Traumatic brain injury and psychiatric diagnoses in veterans seeking outpatient substance abuse treatment. *J Head Trauma Rehabil.* Nov-Dec 2010;25(6):470-479.

Parsons TD, Courtney C, Rizzo AA, Armstrong C, Edwards J, Reger G. Virtual reality paced serial assessment test for neuropsychological assessment of a military cohort. *Stud Health Technol Inform.* 2012;173:331-337.

Pietrzak RH, Goldstein MB, Malley JC, et al. Posttraumatic growth in Veterans of Operations Enduring Freedom and Iraqi Freedom. *J Affect Disord.* Oct 2010;126(1-2):230-235.

Pugh MJV, Knoefel JE, Mortensen EM, Amuan ME, Berlowitz DR, Van Cott AC. New-onset epilepsy risk factors in older veterans. *J Am Geriatr Soc.* Feb 2009;57(2):237-242.

Quigley KS, McAndrew LM, Almeida L, et al. Prevalence of environmental and other military exposure concerns in Operation Enduring Freedom and Operation Iraqi Freedom veterans. *J Occup Environ Med.* Jun 2012;54(6):659-664.

Raymont V, Salazar AM, Krueger F, Grafman J. "Studying injured minds" - the Vietnam head injury study and 40[THIN SPACE]years of brain injury research. *Front Neurol.* 2011;2:15.

Raymont V, Salazar AM, Lipsky R, Goldman D, Tasick G, Grafman J. Correlates of posttraumatic epilepsy 35 years following combat brain injury. *Neurology.* Jul 20 2010;75(3):224-229.

Reiber GE, McFarland LV, Hubbard S, et al. Servicemembers and veterans with major traumatic limb loss from Vietnam war and OIF/OEF conflicts: survey methods, participants, and summary findings. *J Rehabil Res Dev.* 2010;47(4):275-297.

Resnik L, Gray M, Borgia M. Measurement of community reintegration in sample of severely wounded servicemembers. *J Rehabil Res Dev.* 2011;48(2):89-102.

Roberts RJ, Franzen K, Varney NR. Theta bursts, closed head injury, and partial seizure-like symptoms: a retrospective study. *Appl Neuropsychol.* 2001;8(3):140-147.

Rosenbaum M, Najenson T. Changes in life patterns and symptoms of low mood as reported by wives of severely brain-injured soldiers. *J Consult Clin Psychol.* Dec 1976;44(6):881-888.

Russell WR. The development of grand mal after missle wounds of the brain. *Johns Hopkins Med J.* May 1968;122(5):250-253.

Salazar AM, Warden DL, Schwab K, et al. Cognitive rehabilitation for traumatic brain injury: A randomized trial. Defense and Veterans Head Injury Program (DVHIP) Study Group. *Jama.* Jun 21 2000;283(23):3075-3081.

Salinsky M, Spencer D, Boudreau E, Ferguson F. Psychogenic nonepileptic seizures in US veterans. *Neurology.* Sep 6 2011;77(10):945-950.

Sayer NA, Chiros CE, Sigford B, et al. Characteristics and rehabilitation outcomes among patients with blast and other injuries sustained during the Global War on Terror. *Arch Phys Med Rehabil.* Jan 2008;89(1):163-170.

Sayer NA, Cifu DX, McNamee S, et al. Rehabilitation needs of combat-injured service members admitted to the VA Polytrauma Rehabilitation Centers: the role of PM&R in the care of wounded warriors. *Pm R.* Jan 2009;1(1):23-28.

Sayer NA, Nelson D, Nugent S. Evaluation of the Veterans Health Administration traumatic brain injury screening program in the upper Midwest. *J Head Trauma Rehabil.* Nov-Dec 2011;26(6):454-467.

Scholten JD, Sayer NA, Vanderploeg RD, Bidelspach DE, Cifu DX. Analysis of US Veterans Health Administration comprehensive evaluations for traumatic brain injury in Operation Enduring Freedom and Operation Iraqi Freedom Veterans. *Brain Inj.* Sep 2012;26(10):1177-1184.

Stelmack JA, Frith T, Van Koevering D, Rinne S, Stelmack TR. Visual function in patients followed at a Veterans Affairs polytrauma network site: an electronic medical record review. *Optometry.* Aug 2009;80(8):419-424.

Streeter CC, Van Reekum R, Shorr RI, Bachman DL. Prior head injury in male veterans with borderline personality disorder. *J Nerv Ment Dis.* Sep 1995;183(9):577-581.

Sullivan EV, Corkin S. Selective subject attrition in a longitudinal study of head-injured veterans. *J Gerontol.* Nov 1984;39(6):718-720.

Taft CT, Kachadourian LK, Suvak MK, et al. Examining impelling and disinhibiting factors for intimate partner violence in veterans. *J Fam Psychol.* Apr 2012;26(2):285-289.

Taylor BC, Hagel EM, Carlson KF, et al. Prevalence and costs of co-occurring traumatic brain injury with and without psychiatric disturbance and pain among Afghanistan and Iraq War Veteran V.A. users. *Med Care.* Apr 2012;50(4):342-346.

Terrio H, Brenner LA, Ivins BJ, et al. Traumatic brain injury screening: preliminary findings in a US Army Brigade Combat Team. *J Head Trauma Rehabil.* Jan-Feb 2009;24(1):14-23.

Terrio HP, Nelson LA, Betthauser LM, Harwood JE, Brenner LA. Postdeployment traumatic brain injury screening questions: Sensitivity, specificity, and predictive values in returning soldiers. *Rehabil Psychol.* Feb 2011;56(1):26-31.

Van Dyke SA, Axelrod BN, Schutte C. Test-retest reliability of the Traumatic Brain Injury Screening Instrument. *Mil Med.* Dec 2010;175(12):947-949.

Vanderploeg RD, Curtiss G, Schinka JA, Lanham RA, Jr. Material-specific memory in traumatic brain injury: differential effects during acquisition, recall, and retention. *Neuropsychology.* Apr 2001;15(2):174-184.

Vanderploeg RD, Schwab K, Walker WC, et al. Rehabilitation of traumatic brain injury in active duty military personnel and veterans: Defense and Veterans Brain Injury Center randomized controlled trial of two rehabilitation approaches. *Arch Phys Med Rehabil.* Dec 2008;89(12):2227-2238.

Varney NR. Prognostic significance of anosmia in patients with closed-head trauma. *J Clin Exp Neuropsychol.* Mar 1988;10(2):250-254.

Vassallo JL, Proctor-Weber Z, Lebowitz BK, Curtiss G, Vanderploeg RD. Psychiatric risk factors for traumatic brain injury. *Brain Inj.* Jun 2007;21(6):567-573.

Vasterling JJ, Constans JI, Hanna-Pladdy B. Head injury as a predictor of psychological outcome in combat veterans. *J Trauma Stress.* Jul 2000;13(3):441-451.

Walker AE, Blumer D. The fate of World War II veterans with posttraumatic seizures. *Arch Neurol.* Jan 1989;46(1):23-26.

Walker AE, Leuchs HK, Lechtape-Gruter H, Caveness WF, Kretschman C. Life expectancy of head injured men with and without epilepsy. *Arch Neurol.* Feb 1971;24(2):95-100.

Walter KH, Barnes SM, Chard KM. The influence of comorbid MDD on outcome after residential treatment for veterans with PTSD and a history of TBI. *J Trauma Stress.* Aug 2012;25(4):426-432.

Walter KH, Kiefer SL, Chard KM. Relationship between posttraumatic stress disorder and postconcussive symptom improvement after completion of a posttraumatic stress disorder/traumatic brain injury residential treatment program. *Rehabil Psychol.* Feb 2012;57(1):13-17.

Weinstein EA, Lyerly OG. Conversion hysteria following brain injury. *Arch Neurol.* Nov 1966;15(5):545-548.

Weiss GH, Caveness WF, Einsiedel-Lechtape H, McNeel ML. Life expectancy and causes of death in a group of head-injured veterans of World War I. *Arch Neurol.* Dec 1982;39(12):741-743.

Welberg L. Traumatic brain injury: Brain trauma in military veterans. *Nat Rev Neurosci.* Jul 2012;13(7):450.

Wilder Schaaf KP. Polytrauma family needs assessment. *Dissertation Abstracts International: Section B: The Sciences and Engineering.* 2010;71(5-B):3342.

Yaffe K, Vittinghoff E, Lindquist K, et al. Posttraumatic stress disorder and risk of dementia among US veterans. *Arch Gen Psychiatry.* Jun 2010;67(6):608-613.

*Sample includes fewer than 30 mTBI cases*

Akin FW, Murnane OD. Head injury and blast exposure: vestibular consequences. *Otolaryngol Clin North Am.* Apr 2011;44(2):323-334, viii.

Bahraini NH, Brenner LA, Harwood JEF, et al. Utility of the trauma symptom inventory for the assessment of post-traumatic stress symptoms in veterans with a history of psychological trauma and/or brain injury. *Mil Med.* Oct 2009;174(10):1005-1009.

Ben Arzi N, Solomon Z, Dekel R. Secondary traumatization among wives of PTSD and post-concussion casualties: distress, caregiver burden and psychological separation. *Brain Inj.* Aug 2000;14(8):725-736.

Brenner LA, Harwood JEF, Homaifar BY, Cawthra E, Waldman J, Adler LE. Psychiatric hospitalization and veterans with traumatic brain injury: a retrospective study. *J Head Trauma Rehabil.* Nov-Dec 2008;23(6):401-406.

Brenner LA, Ladley-O'Brien SE, Harwood JEF, et al. An exploratory study of neuroimaging, neurologic, and neuropsychological findings in veterans with traumatic brain injury and/or posttraumatic stress disorder. *Mil Med.* Apr 2009;174(4):347-352.

Carr ME, Jr., Masullo LN, Brown JK, Lewis PC. Creatine kinase BB isoenzyme blood levels in trauma patients with suspected mild traumatic brain injury. *Mil Med.* Jun 2009;174(6):622-625.

Chapman JC, Andersen AM, Roselli LA, Meyers NM, Pincus JH. Screening for mild traumatic brain injury in the presence of psychiatric comorbidities. *Arch Phys Med Rehabil.* Jul 2010;91(7):1082-1086.

Chard KM, Schumm JA, McIlvain SM, Bailey GW, Parkinson RB. Exploring the efficacy of a residential treatment program incorporating cognitive processing therapy-cognitive for veterans with PTSD and traumatic brain injury. *J Trauma Stress.* Jun 2011;24(3):347-351.

Classen S, Levy C, Meyer DL, Bewernitz M, Lanford DN, Mann WC. Simulated driving performance of combat veterans with mild traumatic brain injury and posttraumatic stress disorder: a pilot study. *Am J Occup Ther.* Jul-Aug 2011;65(4):419-427.

Davenport ND, Lim KO, Armstrong MT, Sponheim SR. Diffuse and spatially variable white matter disruptions are associated with blast-related mild traumatic brain injury. *Neuroimage.* Feb 1 2012;59(3):2017-2024.

Finkel A. Headaches in soldiers with mild traumatic brain injury - additional data. *Headache.* Sep 2012;52(8):1320.

Finkel AG, Yerry J, Scher A, Choi YS. Headaches in soldiers with mild traumatic brain injury: findings and phenomenologic descriptions. *Headache.* Jun 2012;52(6):957-965.

Homaifar BY, Brenner LA, Gutierrez PM, et al. Sensitivity and specificity of the Beck Depression Inventory-II in persons with traumatic brain injury. *Arch Phys Med Rehabil.* Apr 2009;90(4):652-656.

Homaifar BY, Harwood JE, Wagner TH, Brenner LA. Description of outpatient utilization and costs in group of veterans with traumatic brain injury. *J Rehabil Res Dev.* 2009;46(8):1003-1010.

Huang M-X, Nichols S, Robb A, et al. An automatic MEG low-frequency source imaging approach for detecting injuries in mild and moderate TBI patients with blast and non-blast causes. *Neuroimage.* Jul 2012;61(4):1067-1082.

Huang M-X, Theilmann RJ, Robb A, et al. Integrated imaging approach with MEG and DTI to detect mild traumatic brain injury in military and civilian patients. *J Neurotrauma.* Aug 2009;26(8):1213-1226.

Lew HL, Poole JH, Alvarez S, Moore W. Soldiers with occult traumatic brain injury. *Am J Phys Med Rehabil.* Jun 2005;84(6):393-398.

Matthews SC, Strigo IA, Simmons AN, O'Connell RM, Reinhardt LE, Moseley SA. A multimodal imaging study in U.S. veterans of Operations Iraqi and Enduring Freedom with and without major depression after blast-related concussion. *Neuroimage.* Jan 2011;54 Suppl 1:S69-75.

Peskind ER, Petrie EC, Cross DJ, et al. Cerebrocerebellar hypometabolism associated with repetitive blast exposure mild traumatic brain injury in 12 Iraq war Veterans with persistent post-concussive symptoms. *Neuroimage.* Jan 2011;54 Suppl 1:S76-82.

Roy MJ, Francis J, Friedlander J, et al. Improvement in cerebral function with treatment of posttraumatic stress disorder. *Ann N Y Acad Sci.* Oct 2010;1208:142-149.

Tan G, Fink B, Dao TK, et al. Associations among pain, PTSD, mTBI, and heart rate variability in veterans of Operation Enduring and Iraqi Freedom: a pilot study. *Pain Med.* Oct 2009;10(7):1237-1245.

Trudeau DL, Anderson J, Hansen LM, et al. Findings of mild traumatic brain injury in combat veterans with PTSD and a history of blast concussion. *J Neuropsychiatry Clin Neurosci.* 1998;10(3):308-313.

Wallace DM, Shafazand S, Ramos AR, et al. Insomnia characteristics and clinical correlates in Operation Enduring Freedom/Operation Iraqi Freedom veterans with post-traumatic stress disorder and mild traumatic brain injury: an exploratory study. *Sleep Med.* Oct 2011;12(9):850-859.

Wilkinson CW, Pagulayan KF, Petrie EC, et al. High prevalence of chronic pituitary and target-organ hormone abnormalities after blast-related mild traumatic brain injury. *Front Neurol.* 2012;3:11.

Williams JL, McDevitt-Murphy ME, Murphy JG, Crouse EM. Deployment risk factors and postdeployment health profiles associated with traumatic brain injury in heavy drinking veterans. *Mil Med.* Jul 2012;177(7):789-796.

Wolf GK, Strom TQ, Kehle SM, Eftekhari A. A preliminary examination of prolonged exposure therapy with Iraq and Afghanistan veterans with a diagnosis of posttraumatic stress disorder and mild to moderate traumatic brain injury. *J Head Trauma Rehabil.* Jan-Feb 2012;27(1):26-32.

Writer BW, Schillerstrom JE, Regwan HK, Harlan BS. Executive clock drawing correlates with performance-based functional status in people with combat-related mild traumatic brain injury and comorbid posttraumatic stress disorder. *J Rehabil Res Dev.* 2010;47(9):841-850.

Yurgelun-Todd DA, Bueler CE, McGlade EC, Churchwell JC, Brenner LA, Lopez-Larson MP. Neuroimaging correlates of traumatic brain injury and suicidal behavior. *J Head Trauma Rehabil.* Jul-Aug 2011;26(4):276-289.

### Does not report outcomes that address key questions

McCarroll JE, Gunderson C. 5-year study of incidence rates of hospitalized cases of head injuries in the US Army. *Neuroepidemiology.* 1990;9(6):296-305.

McDonald BC, Saykin AJ, McAllister TW. Functional MRI of mild traumatic brain injury (mTBI): progress and perspectives from the first decade of studies. *Brain imaging behav.* Jun 2012;6(2):193-207.

Schwab KA, Ivins B, Cramer G, et al. Screening for traumatic brain injury in troops returning from deployment in Afghanistan and Iraq: Initial investigation of the usefulness of a short screening tool for traumatic brain injury. *The Journal of Head Trauma Rehabilitation.* Nov-Dec 2007;22(6):377-389.

*Does not meet VA DoD definition for mTBI*

Adams RS, Larson MJ, Corrigan JD, Horgan CM, Williams TV. Frequent binge drinking after combat-acquired traumatic brain injury among active duty military personnel with a past year combat deployment. *J Head Trauma Rehabil.* Sep 2012;27(5):349-360.

Arbisi PA, Polusny MA, Erbes CR, Thuras P, Reddy MK. The Minnesota Multiphasic Personality Inventory-2 Restructured Form in National Guard soldiers screening positive for posttraumatic stress disorder and mild traumatic brain injury. *Psychol Assess.* Mar 2011;23(1):203-214.

Armistead-Jehle P. Symptom validity test performance in U.S. veterans referred for evaluation of mild TBI. *Appl Neuropsychol.* Jan 2010;17(1):52-59.

Bazarian JJ, Zhu T, Blyth B, Borrino A, Zhong J. Subject-specific changes in brain white matter on diffusion tensor imaging after sports-related concussion. *Magn Reson Imaging.* Feb 2012;30(2):171-180.

Booth-Kewley S, Highfill-McRoy RM, Larson GE, Garland CF, Gaskin TA. Anxiety and depression in marines sent to war in iraq and afghanistan. *J Nerv Ment Dis.* Sep 2012;200(9):749-757.

Brenner LA, Ivins BJ, Schwab K, et al. Traumatic brain injury, posttraumatic stress disorder, and postconcussive symptom reporting among troops returning from iraq. *J Head Trauma Rehabil.* Sep-Oct 2010;25(5):307-312.

Brenner LA, Terrio H, Homaifar BY, et al. Neuropsychological test performance in soldiers with blast-related mild TBI. *Neuropsychology.* Mar 2010;24(2):160-167.

Cameron KL, Marshall SW, Sturdivant RX, Lincoln AE. Trends in the incidence of physician-diagnosed mild traumatic brain injury among active duty U.S. military personnel between 1997 and 2007. *J Neurotrauma.* May 2012;29(7):1313-1321.

Clement PF, Kennedy JE. Wechsler Adult Intelligence Scale-third edition characteristics of a military traumatic brain injury sample. *Mil Med.* Dec 2003;168(12):1025-1028.

Dougherty AL, MacGregor AJ, Han PP, Heltemes KJ, Galarneau MR. Visual dysfunction following blast-related traumatic brain injury from the battlefield. *Brain Inj.* 2011;25(1):8-13.

Drake AI, Gray N, Yoder S, Pramuka M, Llewellyn M. Factors predicting return to work following mild traumatic brain injury: A discriminant analysis. *The Journal of Head Trauma Rehabilitation.* Oct 2000;15(5):1103-1112.

Eskridge SL. Combat-related blast injuries: Injury types and outcomes. *Dissertation Abstracts International: Section B: The Sciences and Engineering.* 2012;72(7-B):3929.

Fear N, Jones E, Groom M, et al. Symptoms of post-concussional syndrome are nonspecifically related to mild traumatic brain injury in UK Armed Forces personnel on return from deployment in Iraq: An analysis of self-reported data. *Psychological Medicine.* Aug 2009;39(8):1379-1387.

Ferrier-Auerbach AG, Erbes CR, Polusny MA, Rath CM, Sponheim SR. Predictors of emotional distress reported by soldiers in the combat zone. *J Psychiatr Res.* May 2010;44(7):470-476.

French LM, Lange RT, Iverson GL, Ivins B, Marshall K, Schwab K. Influence of bodily injuries on symptom reporting following uncomplicated mild traumatic brain injury in US military service members. *J Head Trauma Rehabil.* Jan-Feb 2012;27(1):63-74.

Gottshall KR, Gray NL, Drake AI, Tejidor R, Hoffer ME, McDonald EC. To investigate the influence of acute vestibular impairment following mild traumatic brain injury on subsequent ability to remain on activity duty 12 months later. *Mil Med.* Aug 2007;172(8):852-857.

Helfer TM, Jordan NN, Lee RB, Pietrusiak P, Cave K, Schairer K. Noise-induced hearing injury and comorbidities among postdeployment U.S. Army soldiers: April 2003-June 2009. *Am J Audiol.* Jun 2011;20(1):33-41.

Heltemes KJ, Dougherty AL, MacGregor AJ, Galarneau MR. Alcohol abuse disorders among U.S. service members with mild traumatic brain injury. *Mil Med.* Feb 2011;176(2):147-150.

Hoffer ME, Balaban C, Gottshall K, Balough BJ, Maddox MR, Penta JR. Blast exposure: vestibular consequences and associated characteristics. *Otol Neurotol.* Feb 2010;31(2):232-236.

Hoffer ME, Donaldson C, Gottshall KR, Balaban C, Balough BJ. Blunt and blast head trauma: different entities. *Int Tinnitus J.* 2009;15(2):115-118.

Hoge CW, McGurk D, Thomas JL, Cox AL, Engel CC, Castro CA. Mild traumatic brain injury in U.S. Soldiers returning from Iraq. *N Engl J Med.* Jan 31 2008;358(5):453-463.

Ivins BJ, Kane R, Schwab KA. Performance on the Automated Neuropsychological Assessment Metrics in a nonclinical sample of soldiers screened for mild TBI after returning from Iraq and Afghanistan: a descriptive analysis. *J Head Trauma Rehabil.* Jan-Feb 2009;24(1):24-31.

Ivins BJ, Schwab KA, Baker G, Warden DL. Hospital admissions associated with traumatic brain injury in the US Army during peacetime: 1990s trends. *Neuroepidemiology.* 2006;27(3):154-163.

Ivins BJ, Schwab KA, Warden D, et al. Traumatic brain injury in U.S. Army paratroopers: prevalence and character. *J Trauma.* Oct 2003;55(4):617-621.

Ivins BJ. Hospitalization associated with traumatic brain injury in the active duty US Army: 2000-2006. *NeuroRehabilitation.* 2010;26(3):199-212.

Lange RT, Brickell TA, French LM, et al. Neuropsychological Outcome from Uncomplicated Mild, Complicated Mild, and Moderate Traumatic Brain Injury in US Military Personnel. *Arch Clin Neuropsychol.* 2012;27(5):480-494.

Lange RT, Pancholi S, Bhagwat A, Anderson-Barnes V, French LM. Influence of poor effort on neuropsychological test performance in U.S. military personnel following mild traumatic brain injury. *J Clin Exp Neuropsychol.* 2012;34(5):453-466.

Lange RT, Pancholi S, Brickell TA, et al. Neuropsychological Outcome from Blast versus Non-blast: Mild Traumatic Brain Injury in U.S. Military Service Members. *J Int Neuropsychol Soc.* May 2012;18(3):595-605.

Lew HL, Garvert DW, Pogoda TK, et al. Auditory and visual impairments in patients with blast-related traumatic brain injury: Effect of dual sensory impairment on Functional Independence Measure. *J Rehabil Res Dev.* 2009;46(6):819-826.

Luis CA, Vanderploeg RD, Curtiss G. Predictors of postconcussion symptom complex in community dwelling male veterans. *J Int Neuropsychol Soc.* Nov 2003;9(7):1001-1015.

MacGregor AJ, Dougherty AL, Galarneau MR. Injury-specific correlates of combat-related traumatic brain injury in Operation Iraqi Freedom. *The Journal of Head Trauma Rehabilitation.* Jul-Aug 2011;26(4):312-318.

MacGregor AJ, Dougherty AL, Morrison RH, Quinn KH, Galarneau MR. Repeated concussion among U.S. military personnel during Operation Iraqi Freedom. *J Rehabil Res Dev.* 2011;48(10):1269-1278.

MacGregor AJ, Shaffer RA, Dougherty AL, et al. Prevalence and psychological correlates of traumatic brain injury in operation iraqi freedom. *J Head Trauma Rehabil.* Jan-Feb 2010;25(1):1-8.

Macgregor AJ. Physical injury and psychological outcomes among United States combat veterans. *Dissertation Abstracts International: Section B: The Sciences and Engineering.* 2007;68(6-B):3665.

McGuire SA, Marsh RW, Sowin TW, Robinson AY. Aeromedical decision making and seizure risk after traumatic brain injury: longitudinal outcome. *Aviat Space Environ Med.* Feb 2012;83(2):140-143.

Mora AG, Ritenour AE, Wade CE, Holcomb JB, Blackbourne LH, Gaylord KM. Posttraumatic stress disorder in combat casualties with burns sustaining primary blast and concussive injuries. *J Trauma.* Apr 2009;66(4 Suppl):S178-185.

Morgan M, Lockwood A, Steinke D, Schleenbaker R, Botts S. Pharmacotherapy regimens among patients with posttraumatic stress disorder and mild traumatic brain injury. *Psychiatric Services.* Feb 2012;63(2):182-185.

Nelson C, St, Weiser M, Gifford S, Gallimore J, Morningstar A. Knowledge gained from the Traumatic Brain Injury Screen-Implications for treating Canadian military personnel. *Mil Med.* Feb 2011;176(2):156-160.

Olson-Madden JH, Forster JE, Huggins J, Schneider A. Psychiatric diagnoses, mental health utilization, high-risk behaviors, and self-directed violence among veterans with comorbid history of traumatic brain injury and substance use disorders. *J Head Trauma Rehabil.* Sep 2012;27(5):370-378.

Ommaya AK, Ommaya AK, Dannenberg AL, Salazar AM. Causation, incidence, and costs of traumatic brain injury in the U.S. military medical system. *J Trauma.* Feb 1996;40(2):211-217.

Ommaya AK, Salazar AM, Dannenberg AL, Chervinsky AB, Schwab K. Outcome after traumatic brain injury in the U.S. military medical system. *J Trauma.* Dec 1996;41(6):972-975.

Pietrzak RH, Johnson DC, Goldstein MB, Malley JC, Southwick SM. Posttraumatic stress disorder mediates the relationship between mild traumatic brain injury and health and psychosocial functioning in veterans of Operations Enduring Freedom and Iraqi Freedom. *J Nerv Ment Dis.* Oct 2009;197(10):748-753.

Plassman BL, Havlik RJ, Steffens DC, et al. Documented head injury in early adulthood and risk of Alzheimer's disease and other dementias. *Neurology.* Oct 24 2000;55(8):1158-1166.

Polusny MA, Kehle SM, Nelson NW, Erbes CR, Arbisi PA, Thuras P. Longitudinal effects of mild traumatic brain injury and posttraumatic stress disorder comorbidity on postdeployment outcomes in national guard soldiers deployed to Iraq. *Arch Gen Psychiatry.* Jan 2011;68(1):79-89.

Roebuck-Spencer TM, Vincent AS, Twillie DA, et al. Cognitive change associated with self-reported mild traumatic brain injury sustained during the OEF/OIF conflicts. *The Clinical Neuropsychologist.* Apr 2012;26(3):473-489.

Romesser J, Shen S, Reblin M, et al. A preliminary study of the effect of a diagnosis of concussion on PTSD symptoms and other psychiatric variables at the time of treatment seeking among veterans. *Mil Med.* Mar 2011;176(3):246-252.

Rona RJ, Jones M, Fear NT, et al. Mild traumatic brain injury in UK military personnel returning from Afghanistan and Iraq: cohort and cross-sectional analyses. *J Head Trauma Rehabil.* Jan-Feb 2012;27(1):33-44.

Rona RJ, Jones M, Fear NT, Sundin J, Hull L, Wessely S. Frequency of mild traumatic brain injury in Iraq and Afghanistan: are we measuring incidence or prevalence? *J Head Trauma Rehabil.* Jan-Feb 2012;27(1):75-82.

Schneiderman AI, Braver ER, Kang HK. Understanding sequelae of injury mechanisms and mild traumatic brain injury incurred during the conflicts in Iraq and Afghanistan: persistent postconcussive symptoms and posttraumatic stress disorder. *Am J Epidemiol.* Jun 15 2008;167(12):1446-1452.

Skopp NA, Trofimovich L, Grimes J, Oetjen-Gerdes L, Gahm GA. Relations between suicide and traumatic brain injury, psychiatric diagnoses, and relationship problems, active component, U.S. Armed Forces, 2001-2009. *Msmr.* Feb 2012;19(2):7-11.

Theeler BJ, Flynn FG, Erickson JC. Chronic Daily Headache in U.S. Soldiers After Concussion. *Headache.* 2012;52(5):732-738.

Theeler BJ, Flynn FG, Erickson JC. Headaches after concussion in US soldiers returning from Iraq or Afghanistan. *Headache.* Sep 2010;50(8):1262-1272.

Vanderploeg RD, Belanger HG, Curtiss G. Mild traumatic brain injury and posttraumatic stress disorder and their associations with health symptoms. *Arch Phys Med Rehabil.* Jul 2009;90(7):1084-1093.

Vanderploeg RD, Curtiss G, Belanger HG. Long-term neuropsychological outcomes following mild traumatic brain injury. *J Int Neuropsychol Soc.* May 2005;11(3):228-236.

Vanderploeg RD, Curtiss G, Duchnick JJ, Luis CA. Demographic, medical, and psychiatric factors in work and marital status after mild head injury. *J Head Trauma Rehabil.* Mar-Apr 2003;18(2):148-163.

Vasterling JJ, Brailey K, Proctor SP, Kane R, Heeren T, Franz M. Neuropsychological outcomes of mild traumatic brain injury, post-traumatic stress disorder and depression in Iraq-deployed US Army soldiers. *Br J Psychiatry.* Sep 2012;201:186-192.

Wilk JE, Herrell RK, Wynn GH, Riviere LA, Hoge CW. Mild traumatic brain injury (concussion), posttraumatic stress disorder, and depression in U.S. soldiers involved in combat deployments: association with postdeployment symptoms. *Psychosom Med.* Apr 2012;74(3):249-257.

Wilk JE, Thomas JL, McGurk DM, Riviere LA, Castro CA, Hoge CW. Mild traumatic brain injury (concussion) during combat: lack of association of blast mechanism with persistent postconcussive symptoms. *J Head Trauma Rehabil.* Jan-Feb 2010;25(1):9-14.

Yurkiewicz IR, Lappan CM, Neely ET, et al. Outcomes from a US military neurology and traumatic brain injury telemedicine program. *Neurology.* Sep 18 2012;79(12):1237-1243.

# APPENDIX G. PEER REVIEW COMMENTS AND RESPONSES

| Reviewer | Comment | Response |
|---|---|---|
| *Question 1: Are the objectives, scope, and methods for this review clearly described?* | | |
| 1 | No | Noted. |
| 1 | Suggest adding in the background of Executive Summary more rationale (e.g., purpose is understanding OEF/OIF cohort vis-à-vis mTBI for planning etc). | We have made this addition. |
| 1 | Also suggest adding the criteria that were used for inclusion/exclusion at the beginning of the document. | Due to space limitations, we have left reference to inclusion/exclusion criteria in the body of the report and appendices; however, this information will be presented earlier in the planned article publication of the results. |
| 1 | Suggest being more specific when mentioning comparison to controls (e.g., on page 4, were they injured controls, postdeployed controls?) | We have included this information in the data abstraction tables. |
| 2 | No | Noted. |
| 2 | Objectives of the review are clearly described. The scope of this review is clearly described. | Noted. |
| 2 | The methods lack detail. Expectations for reporting methodological detail have grown exponentially over the past few years, and although this would expand the methods section, I highly recommend that this be done. | Noted. We have expanded this discussion. |
| 2 | Specifically, I recommend that the report follow the most recent PRISMA guidelines for reporting systematic reviews. I recognize that this is not primarily an academic document. However, adherence to the PRISMA guidelines would enhance the credibility of the review. | Noted. We have expanded our reporting to be in line with PRISMA guidelines as you suggest. |
| 2 | 1. I assume that no online protocol was published, but if so, that should be reported. | We have updated this information in the report. |
| 2 | 2. Eligibility criteria: The study designs included were mentioned. I have a few questions. Case control studies are not listed in the inclusion criteria. Were case control studies excluded from the search? I assume that case series and case reports were excluded, but this is not explicit. Under the criteria "Timing: No limitations based on timing" – my question – timing of what? Please clarify | Noted. Case control studies were not excluded. Timing has been updated to reflect time since injury. The inclusion criteria have been updated accordingly. |
| 2 | 3. Information Sources: This is well covered. However, if study authors were contacted for additional information, this information should be included. If they were not contacted, it is fine to leave the section as it is. | Correct – no authors were contacted for additional information about studies included in this review. |

| Reviewer | Comment | Response |
|---|---|---|
| 2 | 4. Search: The electronic search is included in appendix A. This is very good. Also, it has become standard practice to clarify that the search was developed by a library scientist experienced in database searches of this sort. It has also recently become recommended practice for a search strategy to be peer reviewed by a second librarian. Was this done? What measures were taken to ensure that the search was comprehensive? | We have added this description of procedures. |
| 2 | 5. Study selection: This section is nicely detailed. Including the study selection form is very useful. Other information to consider adding: What procedures were taken where the PI and the other reviewer disagreed on relevance at the point of abstract screening? What procedures were undertaken where the reviewers disagreed on relevance at the point of full article screening? A detailed definition of TBI is provided in Appendix C. This requires a Mild TBI to have normal CT/MRI. It might be noted in the methods section (or someplace else in the document) that this is not a universally agreed upon criteria – many definitions of MTBI allow for abnormalities on imaging, differentiating these by classifying them as complicated or uncomplicated mild TBI. Of course it is important to adhere to the VA/DoD criteria, but it is a possible point of discrepancy from other criteria that should be explicitly noted. | Thank you. We have included this additional information in the updated report. |
| 2 | 6. Data abstraction: Good tables. It would be useful to have details about the data abstraction process. It has become the standard to have at least two independent data abstractors – was this done? Who did the data abstraction? How was this checked? Again, where data were missing or ambiguous in the report, were authors contacted? It would also be helpful to include study design in the tables. | We have updated the report with this additional information. We chose not to include study design in the tables because the designs were often inaccurately reported in the published studies and because all studies were observational in nature. Specific study design criteria related to quality/ potential for bias were abstracted in the tables (e.g., sample selection, comparison group, etc.) |
| 2 | 7. Quality assessment: In this section, you state that case control and case series designs were included. This should be consistent with the statement of study design inclusion criteria. More details should be provided. Who did the quality assessment? It is standard practice to have two independent quality assessments on each paper, and to report the procedures undertaken when there is no consensus on quality. How (specifically) was the assessment of quality used in the data synthesis process? How specifically was this linked to rating the body of evidence? Who performed this linkage? | This discrepancy has been corrected. We have added this information. |
| 2 | 8. Synthesis: You have provided a reasonable way of grouping the studies and no meta-analysis was conducted – I see this decision as appropriate. However, details about how the synthesis was conducted would be very good to add. This includes who conducted the synthesis, was this discussed in a larger group, were the conclusions agreed to by the working group, and what processes were used to reach agreement. | We have added this information. |

126

| Reviewer | Comment | Response |
|---|---|---|
| 2 | 9. Results: I see a literature flow chart. This is very good. | Noted. |
| 2 | 10. You provide well-formulated summary statements, and in your detailed results sections, you link findings to your citations. But it might also be useful to link findings to the particular studies in your summary statements as well. This is optional, but I present it as worth considering. | Due to the lengthiness of the report, we decided not to link findings to particular studies in the summary section. However, we linked findings in the results section to the citations of included studies should readers be interested in these specifics. |
| 2 | 11. There is no linkage between particular studies and their study quality assessment – or more importantly, their assessed risk of bias. This does not necessarily imply the need for an overall score, and the use of an overall additive score has been widely criticized. But the reader should be able to see which studies have risk of which biases. There is some reference to overall study quality in the sections reporting summary of findings, but most recent standards recommend that this be reported in a more study-specific way. When you say "low quality" – what specifically do you mean? I also wonder whether studies with high risk of bias in their methodological quality can usefully contribute to our knowledge of TBI in the military? | We have updated our description of study quality and risk of bias to specifically describe each study as being of low quality due to the high risk of bias. We have also provided additional cautionary, interpretive statements in the summary section related to the strength of evidence from a body of low quality studies. |
| 2 | 12. Were cross-sectional studies included in sections related to risk or prognostic factors. There is no information provided about the restriction of study designs for particular questions. Obviously, cross-sectional studies are appropriate for questions about prevalence of symptoms, but not for making causal inferences about these symptoms. Could this be clarified in the report? | We have clarified the inclusion of various types of study designs, highlighted findings from the only prospective study, and noted limitations of interpretation based solely on cross sectional studies reporting association rather than causal inferences. |
| 2 | 13. The authors have done a good job in discussing limitations of the literature in the second last section. Would it be useful to be even more specific about biases in the Limitations and Recommendations section? E.g., providing concrete examples of recall bias; of incidence-prevalence bias (where it might exist), etc. | We have added additional discussion of these points. |
| 3 | Yes | Noted. |
| 4 | No | Noted. |
| 4 | 1 The methods section of the Executive Summary is missing important information about inclusion/exclusion criteria and how quality and strength of evidence is rated. This latter point is particularly important as it makes it very difficult for the reader to understand why the authors consider the strength of the evidence to be low. | We have added this information to the executive summary section of the report. |
| 4 | It is also not clear when the authors state that no clear pattern of risk and protective factors emerge whether the studies were designed to look at risk and protective factors. | We have noted this in the discussion. |

| Reviewer | Comment | Response |
|---|---|---|
| 4 | 2. In the Executive Summary Conclusions section (and elsewhere in the report) the authors refer to "objective results" (p.4). It would be helpful if they discussed which results were "objective" and what is meant by "objective". | We have updated this section to describe results not based on self-report. |
| 4 | 3. It is not clear to me why the authors are including the headache intervention study. How is participating in a headache intervention a protective factor? What then is meant by protective factor? Do the authors mean that the sample referred for headache intervention was different than those not referred? Why is that relevant to the KQs? In general, the information presented on this particular study is confusing throughout the report and relevance is not clear. | We have clarified references to this intervention throughout the report. |
| 4 | 4. It is not clear to me why studies focused on biomarkers are included. I do not see how biomarkers are "impairments" (KQ 1) according to any definition of impairment. I do not see how biomarkers address either KQ2A (pre-injury factors) or 2B (post injury factors) if they not include a focus on outcomes, given the way that KQ is worded. How does this study meet criteria for the outcomes listed on p.10? | We agree and have moved information from this section to the discussion rather than including it in the evidence synthesis. |
| 4 | 5. Table 1: I find the mTBI definition column confusing. What do the authors mean by "citation". What do the authors mean when they list "LOC, AOC and PTA" given inclusion criteria requires DOD/VA/ACRM definition of mTBI? A note to the table may help clarify. | We have clarified this column label. |
| 4 | 6. I did not finding tables summarizing strength of evidence per study. This information is particularly important given the conclusions. It would also make it easier for the reader to refer to specific studies when reviewing the report. In the absence of this information, it is difficult to interpret statements like, "Strength of the evidence was low because of ….". If I missed something that was included in the report, I apologize. | We have clarified this information in the text of the report. All included studies were rated as low quality due to high risk of bias, without exception. |
| 4 | 7. Tables 2–6: I would have liked to see the pertinent studies referenced rather than or at least in addition to the number of studies listed in parentheses. Number may not be as important as quality, in my opinion. Question based on Table 2: Did 4 studies find that mean scores for processing speed were within normal limits with possible exceptions of those getting C&Ps and <10 days since injury (p.24)? This is what the Table suggests, unless I am not reading it correctly. | We have referenced individual citations in the text, and due to the low quality rating of all included studies, have not identified individual studies or study quality in the table for reasons of space. You are correct in your interpretation of the presented information in the table. |

| Reviewer | Comment | Response |
|---|---|---|
| 4 | 8. When the authors make statements like "most research reported no significant risk or protective factors," it would be helpful to know the number/percent of studies were looking at risk/protective factors. | We have noted this information in the discussion as an overall commentary on the body of literature given that only one included study was prospective in nature, and the rest were not designed to assess risk/protective factors. We have also clarified these sentences in the report to reflect studies of association rather than implying that studies were designed to assess risk/protective factors. |
| 4 | 9. I do not know that readers who are not neuropsychologists will understand how the authors are distinguishing between cognitive and physical health problems. For example, it may not be clear why visuospatial abilities falls in the cognitive domain but vision is in the physical health results section. It is not clear why the authors review "effort and motivation" at all. It is not clear why studies focused on sleep are in the functional/social outcomes section. I suggest that the authors explicitly describe the rationale for their groupings. | We have provided additional description of these decisions in the report. |
| 4 | 10. In the Executive Summary Limitation section, the authors state that the studies included in the review relied on well-validated assessment tools. Are they classifying the NSI as well-validated? Perhaps this statement can be more precise. | We have made this statement more accurate and non-specific to individual tools. We refer to well-validated assessment tools being a strength of the overall body of literature, and report specific tools in the data abstraction. However, we did not to an individual literature search or other method of assessment to determine validation of each tool used in the included studies. We do also note limitations of some of the tools (e.g., the NSI) used to assess single-item, self-report outcomes. |
| 4 | 11. Service Utilization and Costs: For this section, it does not make sense to me to collapse across Veteran and active duty samples given differences in the healthcare systems. I recommend that the authors clearly state which findings are specific to Veterans using VA and which are specific to active duty. | We have added a clarifying statement noting that all included studies investigated Veterans. |
| 5 | Yes | Noted. |
| 6 | Yes | Noted. |
| 6 | The objectives mention cognitive "disability" as an outcome, but based on the variables examined in the literature, cognitive "deficits" may be a better term. The language regarding mental health outcomes could also be clarified. The objectives mention "symptoms" but the operational definition is later given as diagnoses. However, examination of the measures in the studies included suggests that "symptoms" would be the more accurate term. | We have changed the wording to "deficits." |
| 7 | Yes | Noted. |

| Reviewer | Comment | Response |
|---|---|---|
| 7 | These are well described. | Noted. |
| 8 | Yes | Noted. |
| 8 | Methods and objectives clearly described, but missing some information. There was no discussion of how common features of mTBI, e.g. the presence of comorbidities and multiple TBIs, were handled in inclusion criteria. | We have clarified these criteria in the report. |
| 8 | "Study relevance" was a major factor in exclusion (p.14) but no further information provided on how this criterion was applied. | Study relevance simply implies that the study must provide information included in the KQs and meet inclusion/exclusion criteria. No additional relevance criteria were applied. |
| 8 | Overall weakness in discussion of physical and neuroimaging outcomes. The scope as defined by the key questions does not include imaging or biomarkers as outcomes. It is not clear whether these topics were adequately searched according to the search strategy presented. However, I am not familiar with the abbreviations and formatting used to detail the search strategy, so this was a bit hard to follow. An explanation or reference would be helpful. | We agree and have moved the imaging/biomarker information to the discussion section and removed it from the results/evidence synthesis. |
| 8 | As a general comment, scope is very large and each element (e.g. cognitive effects) could be the subject of a report. | Noted. |
| 9 | Yes | Noted. |
| 9 | The key objectives and methodology are sound. | Noted. |
| 10 | Yes | Noted. |
| 10 | Consider rephrasing to: **Key Question # 1:** For Veterans/Service Members who suffer a mTBI and develop acute and or persistent sequale of mTBI symptoms what is the prevalence of health conditions (e.g. pain, headaches, insomnia, vertigo, or seizure disorder), functional limitations, (e.g. return to work/duty, marital status/family dynamics), cognitive impairment (e.g. attention, concentration or memory) and or associated mental health conditions ( e.g. PTSD, depression or anxiety disorder ). **Key Question # 2:** What factors affect outcomes for Veterans/service members with mTBI? **Key Question 2A:** For Veteran/military populations, are there pre-injury (premorbid) risk factors (e.g., pre-injury mental health factors, genetic factors, or prior concussions) or protective factors ??) that affect outcomes for mTBI? **Key Question 2B:** For Veteran/military populations, are there post-injury risk factors (e.g., PTSD, depression or anxiety) or protective factors that affect outcomes for mTBI? | We have changed the wording of the key questions slightly. |
| 11 | Yes | Noted. |

| Reviewer | Comment | Response |
|---|---|---|
| **2. Is there any indication of bias in our synthesis of the evidence?** | | |
| 1 | No | Noted. |
| 2 | No | Noted. |
| 2 | I don't see an indication of bias, although it is always useful to discuss possible publication bias and how this might impact on the synthesis. However, a synthesis based on highly biased studies can bias a synthesis. Where studies were highly biased (low quality), can it be estimated what direction those methodological flaws would have biased the study's findings? (toward or away from the null, for example). This may impact on the interpretation of study findings. | Noted. We have added these points to the discussion. |
| 3 | No | Noted. |
| 4 | Yes | Noted. |
| 4 | 1. The report states that TBI is THE leading cause of morbidity and disability in OEF/OIF. I do not believe that this is accurate. More important, one needs to distinguish between TBI history and TBI-related disability. The prevalence of TBI-related disability is unknown and some evidence suggests that persistent problems in many individuals who suffered TBI in OEF/OIF result from mental health comorbidities | Noted. We have changed the introductory paragraphs to better reflect these distinctions. |
| 4 | 2. In Executive Summary Conclusions section, the authors state that "It is likely that the prevalence....is largely influenced by factors other than deployment rather than being uniquely associated with mTBI." They do NOT however describe a rationale for this conclusion. This reviewer suggests that the authors clearly build conclusions based on the literature reviewed otherwise the sentence reads like an opinion. The statement in the Executive Summary Conclusions that reads, " ... the most likely exceptions are...evaluation linked with potential compensation" is particularly troubling as it seems to be based on the one study that looked at compensation effects (#34). In the Executive Summary Limitation section the authors state " ...self-reported deficits are more likely to persist for individuals with mTBI particularly when associated with compensation (p.40)." Again, this statement seems too strong if only one study (#34) reviewed looked at compensation effects unless that study was of very high quality | These conclusions are based on consistent findings across Veteran/military and civilian literature, though we agree that the conclusions could have been interpreted as basing conclusions on solely the Veteran/military literature, which would not have been warranted. These concluding statements have been tempered and clarified to more accurately reflect the results available from the body of literature. |

| Reviewer | Comment | Response |
|---|---|---|
| 4 | 3. In the Summary and Discussion section the authors conclude, "The body of research ...suggest that many health consequences resolve within the first few months following injury, if not sooner" (p.49). I am not clear about what evidence they are using the draw that conclusion given the design of the studies reviewed. To which specific studies/findings are the authors referring when they state, "Objective cognitive impairment most often resolves within a few weeks of initial injury."? I suggest that authors be very clear about the findings and studies they are using to make that claim. That claim also seems to be in direct contraction to their statement in the Background section that "TBI is the leading cause of morbidity and disability…" It also contradicts the statement in the Service Utilization/Costs that "The long-term resource needs of recent Iraq and Afghanistan War Veterans who sustained mTBI are likely substantial". (p.52). Why would that be the case? | We have clarified the studies on which these conclusions are based, as sometimes the quotes were in direct reference to the Carroll et al, 2004 review findings that we were summarizing. We have also tempered the introductory statements relating to the potential effects of TBI. |
| 4 | 3. The authors also state in Summary and Discussion, "This report documents that litigation or evaluation for compensation as being a risk factor…(p.49)" Is this the finding based on one study referred to in multiple sections of this report (#34) or are there other studies? The basis for this statement was not clear to me. | This statement was in reference to findings from the Carroll et al, 2004 review, and this citation has been clarified. |
| 5 | Yes | Noted. |
| 5 | The bias has to do with studies included versus excluded. Your criteria are clear and stated on the bottom of page 9, of which the DoD/VA criteria are one operational definition of those criteria. | Noted. |
| 5 | However, the manuscript <u>includes</u> studies that don't meet that criteria because they: | Noted. |
| 5 | (a) include moderates and "unclassified" severity patients [Morrisette, Woodward, Kimbrel, et al, 2011[75], Schiehser, Delis, Filoteo, et al., 2011[35]] or, | Thank you for catching this error. Though this paper reports findings for the mTBI only group separately from those with moderate or unclassified TBI, the specific finding we reported in our review was a combined group finding; therefore, this study has been excluded. |
| 5 | (b) includes those where TBI was not verified ("probably TBI") [Ruff, Riechers, Wang, et al., 2012[32]], or | Though this paper reports some findings for a combined TBI group, the findings that we reported in this review are reported separately for the mTBI only group. |
| 5 | (c) at least as currently written in the tables, state criteria at variance to the DoD/ VA criteria such as the GCS > 13 was used or GCS = 13 (when it should be ≥ 13) [Gaylord, Cooper, Mercado, et al., 2008[21], Cooper, Mercado-Couch, Richfield, et al., 2010[18]]. | You are correct that this was inaccurately stated in the table. It should be ≥ 13, as reported in the article, and therefore these studies remain included. |

| Reviewer | Comment | Response |
|---|---|---|
| 5 | Studies are excluded, that in my view meet the DoD/VA criteria at least as well, if not better, than some of the included studies. Of course I am biased, but I'm referring to my studies: | Noted. We have reviewed all the suggested studies and agree that they provide useful information; however, we have scoped the review to include a specific subset of papers meeting VA/DoD mTBI criteria, and the papers you suggest do not fit within those pre-specified criteria and are therefore not included in the review. |
| 5 | Luis CA, Vanderploeg RD, Curtiss G. Predictors of postconcussion symptom complex in community dwelling male veterans. *J Int Neuropsychol Soc.* Nov 2003;9(7):1001-1015. | Reviewed, not included due to not meeting inclusion criteria. |
| 5 | Vanderploeg RD, Belanger HG, Curtiss G. Mild traumatic brain injury and posttraumatic stress disorder and their associations with health symptoms. *Arch Phys Med Rehabil.* Jul 2009;90(7):1084-1093. | Reviewed, not included due to not meeting inclusion criteria. |
| 5 | Vanderploeg RD, Curtiss G, Belanger HG. Long-term neuropsychological outcomes following mild traumatic brain injury. *J Int Neuropsychol Soc.* May 2005;11(3):228-236. | Reviewed, not included due to not meeting inclusion criteria. |
| 5 | Vanderploeg RD, Curtiss G, Duchnick JJ, Luis CA. Demographic, medical, and psychiatric factors in work and marital status after mild head injury. *J Head Trauma Rehabil.* Mar-Apr 2003;18(2):148-163. | Reviewed, not included due to not meeting inclusion criteria. |
| 5 | Self-report for LOC is not reliable because individuals do not know if they actually had an LOC or simply a memory gap (i.e., PTA). Our studies used alteration of consciousness defined as "loss consciousness or 'black out'". That is, either a self-reported LOC or a self-reported Alteration of consciousness. It is possible, although unlikely, that my studies included a few folks who had moderate injuries. Unlikely because the data was collected in the 1970s at which time those with anything other than a mild TBI would be hospitalized overnight at least, and no subject was hospitalized. In addition, the bias come in because other studies were included that had moderate or "unclassified" TBI severity subjects. | See above comments; we have re-reviewed all noted studies and the inclusion/exclusion criteria have been appropriately applied. Thank you for noting the possible discrepancies as one of the studies was inappropriately included in the first draft of the report and has now been excluded (Morrisette). |
| 5 | None of this would change findings, but my studies do address things the manuscripts says have not been addressed – frequencies of different medical signs and symptoms and psychosocial outcomes, as well as frequencies of neuropsychological impairments, in addition to comparison with an injury control group (groups most other studies do not have) and controlling for comorbid or premorbid medical and mental health conditions. | See above response re: included studies. |

| Reviewer | Comment | Response |
|---|---|---|
| 5 | In addition, core findings of these studies have been replicated in a new sample using criteria that you would likely agree does meet the DoD/VA criteria for mild TBI. This study, also not included, is: Vanderploeg, R.D., Belanger, H.G., Horner, R.D., Spehar, A.M., Powell-Cope, G., Luther, S.L., Scott, S.G., (2012). Health Outcomes Associated With Military Deployment: Mild Traumatic Brain Injury, Blast, Trauma, and Combat Associations in the Florida National Guard. Archives of Physical Medicine and Rehabilitation, 93, 1887-1895. | We have reviewed this study and it does not quite meet VA/DoD criteria, and therefore is not included in the review. |
| 6 | No | Noted. |
| 6 | The selection of studies is straightforward, but given the large number excluded, it might be helpful to summarize in the table of excluded studies, the specific reasons for exclusion. Without knowing how close these studies came to being eligible for inclusion in the paper, it's difficult to assess whether the eligibility criteria themselves may have incidentally introduced a bias. For example, are warzone samples more likely to be excluded than veteran samples due to contextual constraints that somehow limited the information gathered? I'm not suggesting altering the eligibility criteria, but instead suggesting assessing potential "sampling biases" (for inclusion in the review) based on the possible identification of variables consistently associated with failure to use the DoD/VA definition. | We had similar concerns, and this was the rationale for including a table of studies meeting all inclusion criteria except for VA/DoD mTBI definition so that we were transparent about exclusions and readers could examine the list for possible bias in the included/excluded studies. We have also added a table of all the full-text study citations and exclusion codes. |
| 7 | No | Noted. |
| 7 | The review was absent of bias, and was appropriately critical of the lack of rigorous methodology, TBI severity description, and appropriate controls that appear pervasive throughout the literature on TBI in U.S. service members and Veterans. | Noted. |
| 8 | Yes | Noted. |
| 8 | Inclusion criteria introduced biases that should be discussed. Use of VA/DoD criteria for mTBI could time-limit the literature to after 2007; indeed, all included studies were from within the last 3 years. These criteria may also limit to military and VA-affiliated researchers and to US researchers. It is possible that exclusion of studies based on reporting of LOC and PTA led to unnecessary loss of data, as the exact value of these is usually based on self-report and is unreliable. | We agree that any scoping decisions, this one included, introduce potential for bias. This decision was agreed upon by stakeholders for this review in order to obtain the most accurate description of a specific population of interest: Members of the US military/Veterans with mTBI meeting VA/DoD criteria. Therefore, though the report is limited in these ways, the stakeholders agreed that other, broader reports (e.g., the Carroll et al, 2004 WHO mTBI report) could address broader/different questions. In response to your comment, we have broadened the discussion of this point in the discussion. |

| Reviewer | Comment | Response |
|---|---|---|
| 8 | The requirement for an mTBI sample size of at least 30 will bias the type of outcome measures that are used. Because of expense and other limitations, few neuroimaging studies will fulfill this requirement. Large studies can be limited in the ability to perform in-depth testing, and so the report may be biased toward less sensitive questionnaire data and easier-to-administer testing protocols (e.g. RBANS is a screening measure designed for dementia). Large studies also may bias away from presentation of individual results, which as you note, can be informative. Few objective evaluations of physical outcomes (e.g. audiology) were included, which severely limits interpretation of this domain. | We agree, and have moved the neuroimaging information to the discussion section because of the likelihood that it is not comprehensive since we did not design the search to focus on these outcomes. We have also now added a table of excluded studies so that authors can review studies that were excluded based on sample size to gather additional information as needed. |
| 8 | Many studies served as sources across outcome domains (e.g. Nelson et al., 2012). This could potentially perpetuate any biases or limitations present in the single study across domains (e.g. recruitment setting, inadequate power). | We agree and have noted this limitation in the discussion. |
| 9 | No | Noted. |
| 10 | No | Noted. |
| 11 | No | Noted. |
| **3. Are there any published or unpublished studies that we may have overlooked?** | | |
| 1 | Yes | Noted. |
| 1 | Cohen, Suri, Amick, & Yan, 2012 (published in Work) | This study does not meet our inclusion criteria because of unclearly reported definition of mTBI and because results are not reported separately for those with mTBI versus moderate/severe TBI. |
| 2 | No | Noted. |
| 2 | Not that I can think of. | Noted. |
| 3 | Yes | Noted. |
| 3 | Scholten et al, Analysis of US Veterans Health Administration comprehensive evaluations for traumatic brain injury in Operation Enduring Freedom and Operation Iraqi Freedom Veterans. Brain Inj 2012 | We have reviewed this study and it does not meet inclusion criteria due to the mTBI definition used to define the cohort of participants. |
| 4 | Yes | Noted. |
| 4 | Have the authors reviewed the CBO report: The Veterans Health Administration's Treatment of PTSD and Traumatic Brain Injury Among Recent Combat Veterans? | We have reviewed this report and agree that though it provides important information and guidance, it does not meet our criteria for inclusion in this review. |
| 5 | Yes | Noted. |

| Reviewer | Comment | Response |
|---|---|---|
| 5 | Vanderploeg, R.D., Belanger, H.G., Horner, R.D., Spehar, A.M., Powell-Cope, G., Luther, S.L., Scott, S.G., (2012). Health Outcomes Associated With Military Deployment: Mild Traumatic Brain Injury, Blast, Trauma, and Combat Associations in the Florida National Guard. Archives of Physical Medicine and Rehabilitation, 93, 1887-1895. | We have reviewed this study and agree that though it provides important information, it does not meet VA/DoD mTBI definitional criteria and is therefore not included in this review. |
| 6 | Yes | Noted. |
| 6 | To my knowledge, the report captures all of the military/military veteran studies. However, in the discussion of meta-analytic studies from the civilian literature, it would be important to balance the discussion with the Pertab et al., meta-analysis that re-analyzes data from previous meta-analytic studies and reveals a potential qualification of prior findings. | This review has been added to the report. |
| 7 | Yes | Noted. |
| 7 | JRRD has recently come out with a TBI sensory and communications disorders edition (Vol. 49, Issue 7, 2012). Even though this journal is published after Oct. 3, 2012, these articles cover deployment-related experiences (e.g., blast, TBI), and associations with the following senses, conditions, and patterns: vestibular, visual, auditory, pain, PTSD, and referrals. This compendium fits well with the focus of the synthesis. | Thank you for this suggestion. We have reviewed all studies from this special issue none meet criteria for inclusion in this report. |
| 7 | Other published studies that were not included, though would be excluded for not meeting mTBI criteria, are:

1. Iverson, K. M., Hendricks, A., Kimerling, R., Krengel, M., Meterko, M., Stolzmann, K., Baker, E., Pogoda, T.K., Vasterling, J., & Lew, H.L. (2011). Psychiatric diagnoses and neurobehavioral symptom severity among OEF/OIF VA patients with deployment-related TBI. Women's Health Issues, 2(4S), S210-S217. | We have reviewed this study and agree that though it provides important information, it does not meet VA/DoD criteria and is therefore not included in this review. |
| 7 | 2. Lew, H.L., Kraft, M., Pogoda, T.K., Amick, M.M., Woods, P., & Cifu, D.X. (2011). Prevalence and Characteristics of Driving Difficulties in Operation Enduring Freedom/Operation Iraqi Freedom Combat Returnees. JRRD, 48(8), 913-926. | We have reviewed this study and agree that though it provides important information, it does not meet VA/DoD criteria and is therefore not included in this review. |
| 7 | 3. Lew, H. L., Pogoda, T.K., Baker, E., Meterko, M., Stolzmann, K.L., Cifu, D.X., Amara, J.H. & Hendricks, A.M. (2011). Prevalence of dual sensory impairment and its association with traumatic brain injury and blast exposure in OEF/OIF Veterans. Journal of Head Trauma & Rehabilitation, 26(6):489-96. | We have reviewed this study and agree that though it provides important information, it does not meet VA/DoD criteria and is therefore not included in this review. |
| 7 | 4. Hendricks AM, Amara J, Baker E, Charns MP, Gardner JA, Iverson KM, et al. (in press) Screening for mild traumatic brain injury in OEF-OIF deployed US military: an empirical assessment of VHA's experience. Brain Injury | We were not able to obtain a copy of this study for review. |
| 8 | Yes | Noted. |

| Reviewer | Comment | Response |
|---|---|---|
| 8 | Luethcke et al. 2010. Comparison of Concussive Symptoms, Cognitive Performance, and Psychological Symptoms Between Acute Blast-Versus Nonblast-Induced Mild Traumatic Brain Injury. Journal of the International Neuropsychological Society (2011), 17, 36–45. | We reviewed this study and it did not meet inclusion criteria. |
| 8 | Terrio, et al. 2009 Traumatic Brain Injury Screening: Preliminary Findings in a US Army Brigade Combat Team. J Head Trauma Rehabil Vol. 24, No. 1, pp. 14–23. | We reviewed this study and it did not meet inclusion criteria. |
| 8 | Caplan et al. 2010 The Structure of Postconcussive Symptoms in 3 US Military Samples. J Head Trauma Rehabil Vol. 25, No. 6, pp. 447–458. | We reviewed this study and it did not meet inclusion criteria. |
| 8 | Cockerham, 2009. Eye and visual function in traumatic brain injury. J Rehab Research Dev Volume 46, Number 6, 2009 Pages 811–818. | We reviewed this study and it did not meet inclusion criteria. |
| 8 | Akin and Murnane, 2011. Head Injury and Blast Exposure: Vestibular Consequences. Otolaryngol Clin N Am 44 (2011) 323–334. | We reviewed this study and it did not meet inclusion criteria. |
| 8 | Pogoda et al., 2012. Multisensory Impairment Reported by Veterans with and without Traumatic Brain Injury History. J Rehab Research Dev Volume 49, Number 7 Pages 971–984. | This study has been included in the report. Thank you for the suggestion. |
| 8 | Vasterling, et al. 2012. Neuropsychological outcomes of mild traumatic brain injury, post-traumatic stress disorder and depression in Iraq-deployed US Army soldiers· Br J Psychiatry 201, 186-192 | We reviewed this study and it did not meet inclusion criteria. |
| 8 | Schneibel et al., 2012 Altered brain activation in military personnel with one or more traumatic brain injuries following blast. J Int Neuropsychol Soc. 2012 Jan;18(1):89-100 | We have moved the discussion of imaging and biomarkers to the discussion section of the report since it falls outside the scope of our key questions. |
| 8 | Morey et al., 2012 Effects of chronic mild traumatic brain injury on white matter integrity in Iraq and Afghanistan war veterans. Hum Brain Mapp. 2012 Jun 15 | We have moved the discussion of imaging and biomarkers to the discussion section of the report since it falls outside the scope of our key questions. |
| 8 | Yurgelon-Todd, et al.,2011. Neuroimaging Correlates of Traumatic Brain Injury and Suicidal Behavior J Head Trauma Rehabil Vol. 26, No. 4, pp. 276–289 | We reviewed this study and it did not meet inclusion criteria. |
| 8 | Sponheim, 2011. Evidence of disrupted functional connectivity in the brain after combat-related blast injury. NeuroImage 54 (2011) S21–S29 | We have moved the discussion of imaging and biomarkers to the discussion section of the report since it falls outside the scope of our key questions. |
| 8 | Peskind et al., 2011. Cerebrocerebellar hypometabolism associated with repetitive blast exposure mild traumatic brain injury in 12 Iraqi war Veterans with persistent post-concussive symptoms. NeuroImage 54 (2011) S76–S82. | We reviewed this study and it did not meet inclusion criteria. |
| 9 | Not aware of any that have been excluded that meet criteria for inclusion. Please see below regarding Vision data. | Noted. |
| 10 | Yes | Noted. |

| Reviewer | Comment | Response |
|---|---|---|
| 10 | Cooper DB et al. Relationship between mechanism of injury and neurocognitive functioning in OEF/OIF service members with mild traumatic brain injuries. Mil Med. 2012 Oct;177(10):1157-60. | This study has been included in the report. Thank you for the suggestion. |
| 10 | Scholten JD et al. Analysis of US Veterans Health Administration comprehensive evaluations for traumatic brain injury in Operation Enduring Freedom and Operation Iraqi Freedom Veterans. Brain Inj. 2012;26(10):1177-84. | We have reviewed this study and it does not meet inclusion criteria due to the mTBI definition used to define the cohort of participants. |
| 10 | Bryan CJ, et al. Loss of Consciousness, Depression, Posttraumatic Stress Disorder, and Suicide Risk Among Deployed Military Personnel With Mild Traumatic Brain Injury. J Head Trauma Rehabil. 2012 Oct 16. | This study has been added to the included studies for this report. Thank you for the suggestion. |
| 11 | Yes | Noted. |
| 11 | During an earlier call you had mentioned that another group (I believe IOM) was conducting a review of mTBI literature. It would be helpful to note this since non-Veteran studies were not included in the literature review and could have been aggregated to be the comparison to the Veteran based studies. | Agreed. The WHO group lead by Dr. Linda Carroll is updating the 2004 mTBI prognosis review, and we have included this information in our report for reader reference. |
| **4. Please write additional suggestions or comments below. If applicable, please indicate the page and line numbers from the draft report.** | | |
| 1 | On page 26, please define "old learning." More specificity in general would be helpful (so for example, for 'memory studies', were delayed recall, trial-by-trial learning, recognition all examined? On page 48 in the summary of results, to what type of control groups were mTBI compared? On page 53, suggest adding the number of control groups were mTBI compared? On page 54, suggest being judicious with the use of the word "persistent" since it is unclear if symptoms persist in the longitudinal sense. | We have changed "old learning" to be "language abilities and general fund of verbal knowledge." We have included additional information on specific tests and on comparison groups in the appendix tables. We have added a statement in the discussion relating to future research of the number of TBIs. We have clarified and limited use of the term persistent throughout the report. |
| 2 | Page 49, Where other reviews are cited, it would be useful to explicitly indicate what year they were published, since early systematic reviews might simply be outdated. The study citation is included, of course, but inclusion of the year of publication in the body of this section would highlight that point. | We have included the year in text in this section. |
| 3 | Overall, an excellent evidence review. | Noted. Thank you. |
| 3 | It should be emphasized for all domains that major shortcomings in the literature are the lack of non-mTBI comparison groups and lack of adequate pre-mTBI (premorbid) data. | Agreed, and we have added this point to the discussion. |
| 3 | In section on mental disorders, some controlled civilian studies do show higher rates of mental disorders after mTBI compared with non-TBI controls (e.g., Fann et al, Arch Gen Psychiatry 2004). Presence of prior psychiatric conditions is a major risk factor. Data from this same cohort showed higher health care utilization among those with mTBI compared with non-TBI controls (Rockhill et al, J Neurotrauma 2012). | We have clarified that some civilian literature indicates higher rates of mental disorders after mTBI, as noted in the Carroll et al 2004 review. |

| Reviewer | Comment | Response |
|---|---|---|
| 4 | Below I provide specific comments about organization and note some areas where the terms used where not clear to me. Please disregard if not helpful in this efforts to finalize the report. | Thank you for the suggestions. Some will be included in this report, though some will be included in the planned article publication rather than in this full report. |
| 4 | 1. I suggest that the authors orient the reader at the beginning to their overall approach to summarizing the findings. It took this reviewer a few reads to understand how the authors were presenting the material. It was a bit confusing to me to read the summary before the sections describing findings per domain (i.e., summary of cognitive functioning in general before description in each cognitive domain). Sometimes the summaries seem completely unnecessary because only one study is reviewed. In general, there was considerable repetition because of the structure of this report, which made the report difficult to read. It takes several reads to know what is new information versus a restating of what has already been summarized. | Because some parts of this report are purposely repetitive (e.g., the executive summary), we plan to make the suggested change for the published article. |
| 4 | 2. This reviewer suggests the authors state reason time since injury is important rather than assuming the reader already has this information. | Noted, and this has been added. |
| 4 | 3. To help the reader understand the "cognitive function" section, I suggest the authors tell the reader that x# studies are based on neuropsychological testing and briefly explain. It would be helpful to have an appendix in which the function each test assesses is described – otherwise, I am not sure how helpful it is to list measures/acronyms in Appendix E. I did not find it useful to have the names of the tests listed in the text – in fact, I think it makes the narrative harder to read. | We have made some of these changes, including shortening the acronyms listed in the results section of the report. |
| 4 | 4. In the Summary of Findings for Cognitive Function Results the author state that "standardized scores are scores associated with impairment below a certain cutoff." This is not quite right and I do not think the sentence expresses what they intend it to. | We have corrected this sentence. |
| 4 | 5. It is confusing when the authors state that risk factors include "LOC and PTA" or the like, given that they are using the DoD/VA/ACRM definition of mTBI. As opposed to what? | We have clarified that LOC and PTA were compared to just alteration of consciousness. |
| 4 | 6. It would be more accurate on p.39 to state that the PCL scores suggest clinically significant *symptoms* rather than "impairment" as stated in the report | We have chosen to use the term impairment across measures to use similar terminology describing scores above a clinically significant cutoff. |
| 4 | 7. The term "TBI sequelae" as used here is confusing. For example, on p. 28 the authors state that one study reported "...based on mTBI with LOC and PTA compared to those with mTBI who did not have these immediate sequelae." What does this mean? If these individuals did not have these "sequelae", how was mTBI determined? This is probably a matter of simple clarification. | We have changed this sentence to clarify. |

| Reviewer | Comment | Response |
|---|---|---|
| 4 | 8. Summary and Conclusions: This section is largely devoted to discussion of the civilian literature. The subsection on Physical Health Outcomes (p.49) does not even discuss the Veteran/military studies. I suggest switching the focus so that the authors primarily discuss the literature they reviewed for this report. | Noted. We have updated the physical health section to focus the discussion on a comparison. |
| 4 | 9. It seems to me that references are used inconsistently. Why are there no references for the summaries? Why are the "one study" referred to on p. 26 and the "single studies" on .34 not referenced What are the "some studies" (p.30 that found better cognitive function for those not evaluated in forensic settings? I thought there was just one study that examined this issue (#34). In some sections, it is very difficult to identify which studies are forming the basis of the authors' conclusions. | Noted. We have made the suggested corrections to text. The format for this report is such that summaries do not contain citations; however, citations will be used consistently throughout the published article. |
| 4 | 10. Note that PTSD is an AXIS I disorder (p.35). I do not understand the statement, "Finally, though many individual studies...general association between specific mental health outcomes with other mental health diagnoses and symptoms". | We have clarified that some studies looked at only PTSD, some examined "any Axis I disorder" which would include PTSD. We have clarified the confusing sentence. |
| 5 | 1. A statement is made without any supporting reference, that I do not believe the literature supports. Page 1: "TBI is the leading cause of morbidity and disability among OEF/OIF service members." I'm not sure about "morbidity" (but I think chronic pain and mental health are higher), but I'm quite sure there is no evidence to support the "disability" claim. This statement is repeated several times throughout the manuscript. | This has been corrected throughout the manuscript. |
| 5 | 2. Page 2 bottom (and elsewhere) "One or more studies have found . . . [problems in those] experiencing loss or alteration of consciousness at the time of the injury." It seems to me that everyone included in every study meets this criteria because that is the criteria for TBI. So, that statement it seems problematic. If all studies had all subjects with an immediate event-related "loss or alteration of consciousness" how can "loss or alteration of consciousness at the time of injury" be a unique factor? | We have clarified that this refers only to patients who have PTA but not LOC or AOC, as described by the primary study authors. |
| 5 | 3. Page 3 (an elsewhere): If you include my studies (or the one you inadvertently omitted because it was recently published), the statement "Similar to objective cognitive results, prevalence of self-reported cognitive deficits was not reported in the included studies" would be inaccurate. | We have updated all summary statements to reflect the final list of articles meeting inclusion criteria. |

| Reviewer | Comment | Response |
|---|---|---|
| 5 | 4. Page 5: The statement "… self-reported deficits are more likely to persist for individuals with mTBI" is inaccurate. There is a difference between "persistence of symptoms" and "symptoms reported in the chronic phase" which may come-and-go or wax-and-wane. Studies have not demonstrated persistence. What they have demonstrated is problems/symptoms reported in the post-acute or chronic phase. The studies do not document that these began at the time of the mTBI and persisted over time to the time of assessment. Other civilian literature clearly documents that symptoms and problems are not persistent, but rather that they come-and-go or wax-and-wane, but are generally higher in frequency in mild TBI subjects. We don't know if they were also higher prior to the mild TBI but we do know that they are not persistent. | We have made this change throughout the report. |
| 5 | 5. The term "Language and Old Learning" is a term no one uses, and as a result is confusing. Initially I thought you were referring to "Verbal Learning and Memory". I would suggest using the term "Language Abilities and General Fund of Verbal Knowledge" or something like that. | Thank you for this suggestion. We have made this change. |
| 5 | 6. Throughout the review you refer to "statistical significance" or lack thereof. However, effect size would seem to better capture the important issue. If sample sizes are somewhat small (or there are is lot of variability across participants) a moderate effect size could be non-significant, but a moderate effect size would be clinically important. | We agree entirely. We report effect sizes in the tables whenever available; however, authors frequently did not report effect sizes or data with which effect sizes could be calculated. |
| 5 | 7. A similar point to that above, is that studies may compare a mild TBI group to a non-mild TBI control group and find differences (as some studies did). However, those two groups may differ on other important factors as well that could explain group differences (e.g., education, race, age, degree of comorbid mental health or medical health conditions). It seems to me that you would want to address this issue if you can for those studies that reported group differences. An example of this is on the bottom of page 26. | Agreed. We highlighted any statistical adjustment or other adjustment for variation across groups in the text and tables; unfortunately, most studies did not provide this information, and this lack of adjustment for potential confounders is a contributing factor to the low study quality ratings for this body of literature. |
| 5 | 8. Page 36: The term "associated with mTBI" is used in talking about mental health disorders and symptoms. This implies some actual association, when it is more likely that they are simply comorbid factors both due to deployment-related (or life-related) experiences that are risk factors for both mTBI and comorbid mental health conditions.<br>-- I would suggest using the term "comorbid" rather than "associated". | We have made this change to the paper. |

| Reviewer | Comment | Response |
|---|---|---|
| 6 | Studies reporting mean cognitive performance scores are criticized within the report because they cannot provide prevalence estimates of impairment. However, the implication that report of percentage of participants scoring below an impairment cut-off or below a certain standard score would yield a good prevalence estimate of cognitive impairment does not take into account the premorbid cognitive abilities of participants. Clinically relevant cognitive impairment is typically thought of as an intra-individual decline. Scores normally thought of as below average may not indicate acquired impairment but instead reflect the innate potential of the individuals; similarly, above average scores may indicate a cognitive decline (i.e., impairment) in an individual with superior cognitive potential. Thus, the suggestion in the report does not go far enough. To best estimate the prevalence of cognitive impairment following a TBI, prospective, longitudinal measurement would be necessary. This is typically not feasible, but the report should nevertheless avoid implications that use of normative data without regard to the individual's baseline potential would yield accurate prevalence estimates of cognitive decline. The paper states this in the Summary and Discussion section, but it is also important to mention it earlier when discussion impairment cut-offs based on standardized scores. | Noted. We have included this discussion both within the section on cognitive outcomes, and within the discussion section. |
| 7 | Overall comments: The synthesis was very well written and took a comprehensive approach to examining the extant literature on mTBI in U.S. service members and military. The synthesis was inconsistent with respect to its use of citations in the text, and its repetition of acronyms and abbreviations. Other editorial and substantive comments (line numbers not included in reviewed drafts): | Noted. Thank you. |
| 7 | P. 1, Background: OEF/OIF should be defined. Also, what about OND? | This change has been made. No studies reported outcomes for OND Veterans and the information we describe in the background is specific to OEF/OIF Veterans. |
| 7 | P. 1 - Methods: Define WHO | This change has been made. |
| 7 | P. 3 - define LOC, PTA | This change has been made. |
| 7 | P. 3 - First introduction of NSI – Neurobehavioral Symptoms (no S) Inventory | This change has been made. |
| 7 | P. 3 – second to last paragraph, two instances of "reported that" – delete one | This change has been made. |
| 7 | P.3 – second to last paragraph – "mTBI)." ß no reference to an open parentheses, so delete the ) | This change has been made. |
| 7 | P.4—define DTI, MRI | This change has been made. |

142

| Reviewer | Comment | Response |
|---|---|---|
| 7 | P.5 – last paragraph: the recommendation to include imaging results is noted; however, such a recommendation is not feasible in terms of equipment, manpower, participant willingness to participate (might lead to biased self-selection), timing, and costs. This recommendation also needs to be reconciled with the VA/DoD Clinical Practice Guidelines (see excerpt below). Though, the point is taken that if imaging studies, especially functional fMRI or DTI, were performed more frequently, then perhaps there would be notable distinctions between "normal" and "mild TBI" states.<br><br>From: VA/DoD (p. 16) | Noted, and we have changed this recommendation slightly to be more consistent with this comment. |
| 7 | In addition to traditional imaging studies, other imaging techniques such as functional magnetic resonance imaging, diffusion tensor imaging, positron emission tomography scanning; electrophysiological testing such as electroencephalography; and neuropsychological or other standardized testing of function have been used in the evaluation of persons with TBIs, but are not considered in the currently accepted criteria for measuring severity at the time of the acute injury outlined in Table A -1 | Noted, and the criteria presented are consistent with the VA/DoD criteria. |
| 7 | Abbreviations Table: There were some abbreviations throughout the text that were not "formally" defined before their first use, so these are included along with others: (a) AOC = Alteration of consciousness/mental state [5] (based on VA/DOD guidelines) p.5; (b) BAMC (last row) = Brooke Army Medical Center, p. 16; (c) C&P = Compensation & Pension , p. 21; (d) CTE = Chronic Traumatic Encephalopathy, p. 10; (e) EFP = Explosively formed penetrator (?) – used on p. 17 – define; (f) mBIAS – "symptoms" misspelled, p. 6; (g) NSI = I = Inventory, p. 6; (h) PI = Principal Investigator, p. 9 (or just say "Principal Investigator on p. 9); (i) VHA = Veterans Health Administration (like on p. 8), p. 7; (j) For SCID, indicate Axis I, not Axis 1, p. 7; (k) Define/include VACO and PM&R, as introduced on p. 8; (l) define WHO on p. 7 (mentioned on p. 8) | These changes have been made. |
| 7 | P. 8 – cite the studies from which the "12 to 23 percent" are derived. Also consider citing Hendricks et al. (in press, Brain Injuries), who examined VA comprehensive TBI evaluation (CTBIE) data and found: "In the study population, 21.6% screened positive for potential TBI and 54.6% of these had an electronic record of a CTBIE. Of those with CTBIE records, evaluators confirmed TBI in 57.7%, yielding a best estimate that 6.8% of all those screened were confirmed to have TBI." | This citation has been added. |
| 7 | P. 8 – second paragraph: "fame" should be "frame" | This change has been made. |

| Reviewer | Comment | Response |
|---|---|---|
| 7 | P.8 – second paragraph: "factors unique to combat deployments." I would take out "combat," (maybe replace with "military," but not sure if that's necessary), since deployment-related conditions (e.g., noise in the general military environment), separate from combat, may uniquely account for experiencing post-concussive symptoms. Plus, since women are restricted from some combat roles, the use of "combat" here may minimize what women potentially experience. | This change has been made. |
| 7 | P. 8 – misplaced semi-colon in second paragraph, | This change has been made. |
| 7 | P. 8 abbreviate "Veterans Health Administration" as VHA; | This change has been made. |
| 7 | P. 8 Define PM&R and VACO | This change has been made. |
| 7 | P. 9 Search strategy – can now call it "mTBI" | This change has been made. |
| 7 | P. 9 Last paragraph – why not include "post-traumatic amnesia" along with AOC, LOC? | This change has been made. |
| 7 | P. 9 – last paragraph, discussion about "severity of sequelae" gets a little confusing, because TBI sequelae can be defined as either AOC, LOC, or PTA (which the reader might be primed for, since there was just discussion about these in the previous sentence), or TBI residual symptoms (e.g., headache, vestibular, pain, auditory, visual, etc. impairment). I don't know if "the Severity of sequelae" sentence needs to be here, but I understand that it makes the point that very specific criteria are used to categorize TBI severity, and it's important to note that the severity of mental/physical symptoms following a TBI event are not used to classify severity. I would replace "sequelae" with "symptoms," and then provide a few NSI-22 symptoms to orient the reader. It might also be helpful to briefly state severity is based on the duration of LOC, AOC, or PTA. You can then list the criteria (e.g., LOC < 30 min), or refer to the reader to a more detailed description, as you currently do. | This change has been made. |
| 7 | P. 10 Identify DoD in first paragraph | This change has been made. |
| 7 | P. 10 – identify CTE in "Outcomes" paragraph | This change has been made. |
| 7 | P. 14, Figure 1: Bullet points in the last box to the right would help the criteria stand out more. | We left out bullet points for space reasons. |
| 7 | P. 15, Table 1: Barnes et al., spell out "medical" | We have corrected this mistake. |
| 7 | P. 16-17 Cooper, Mercado-Couch, et al. – BAMC should be defined earlier (e.g., in the Cooper et al. citation above it in the table); Should American "College" be "Congress?"; Was not clear about 10 participants excluded due to PTA suggesting a more severe TBI... Is it that the duration of PTA was longer than the criteria for mTBI, as specified by ACRM? | This change has been made. |

| Reviewer | Comment | Response |
|---|---|---|
| 7 | P. 17 Drag et al., define "C and P," also, in mTBI definition, why not just call it "AOC?" | This change has been made. |
| 7 | P. 17 Gaylord et al., American College or Congress?; defined "EFP," as previously noted. | This change has been made. |
| 7 | P. 18 Gordon et al., Time since Injury – define unit of time. | This change has been made. |
| 7 | P. 18, Kennedy, Leal et al., last column, just say MVA instead of spelling it out | This change has been made. |
| 7 | P. 19 MacDonald et al., use "TBI" consistently – sometimes it's spelled out (see first and last columns) | This is a quote so it is spelled out as in the original text. |
| 7 | P. 19 Morrisette et al., spell "through," not "thru." | This change has been made. |
| 7 | P. 19, Nelson et al., reference 34: define what "forensic" context is. | This change has been made. |
| 7 | P. 20, Patil et al., Based on "VA"/DoD Consensus definition (reversed as written). | This change has been made. |
| 7 | P. 20 Ruff, Riechers et al., "Department of CVAMC" needs editing; also, in description for three groups of Veterans, for the first two indicate "deployment-related" LOC? Not sure what "combat Veterans without "LOC" means – is this a control group or did they have AOC or PTA?; In the mTBI definition column, not sure what the definition is referring to – did Veterans have to have LOC or AOC following the TBI, PLUS PTA? | These changes have been made. |
| 7 | P. 21 Schiesher et al., mTBI definition column – delete © | This change has been made. |
| 7 | P. 21 Spencer et al., C&P needs to be defined earlier | This change has been made. |
| 7 | P. 21 Swick et al., Combat Veterans diagnosed, not "diagnoses" | This change has been made. |
| 7 | P. 21 Theeler et al., mTBI definition column – use DVBIC acronym | This change has been made. |
| 7 | P. 23 Third from last paragraph – can abbreviate LOC and AOC – make clear, if this is the case, that participants demonstrated better overall cognitive functioning "post-intervention?" | This change has been made. |
| 7 | P. 23 – wasn't clear in 2nd to last paragraph – second line: Should this be "NOT" reported, or should "NOT" be deleted? | We have clarified this sentence. |
| 7 | P. 24, processing speed row, Key Question #1 column, not sure why "possible" exceptions is there – delete that word? | This change has been made. |
| 7 | P. 26, first paragraph – could you cite the 7 studies here? | We are providing summary paragraphs without citations for each section, which are followed by the cited results sections by key question. This will be consolidated for the published article version of the report. |

| Reviewer | Comment | Response |
|---|---|---|
| 7 | P. 26, first paragraph, 2nd line, instead of "with" TBI, replace "with" with "experienced" or indicate "with mTBI history." Also make this correction in Key Question 2 paragraph, first line. | This change has been made. |
| 7 | P. 26, Visuospatial abilities, first sentence, cite the 5 studies here. | We are providing summary paragraphs without citations for each section, which are followed by the cited results sections by key question. This will be consolidated for the published article version of the report. |
| 7 | P. 26, last full paragraph: Just give the abbreviations/acronyms, no need to spell out the neuropsychological test names. | This change has been made. |
| 7 | P. 27, first paragraph, 3rd line: instead of saying "significant correlations," indicate directionality, since it seems like visuospatail abilities and MH conditions would be negatively correlated. | This change has been made. |
| 7 | P. 27, first "Memory" paragraph, mid-way through, again report direction of association. | This change has been made. |
| 7 | P. 27, Key Question 1 paragraph: just report abbreviations | This change has been made. |
| 7 | P. 27, Key Question 1 paragraph, 5th from last row, use "longer" instead of "much more." | This change has been made. |
| 7 | P. 27, second to last row, use (C&P) for compensation and pension, since this would have been introduced previously. | This change has been made. |
| 7 | P. 28, 1st paragraph, second from last row: Use LOC and PTA instead of spelling them out. | This change has been made. |
| 7 | P. 28, Attention/Concentration paragraph, cite the 7 studies after mentioning them. | We are providing summary paragraphs without citations for each section, which are followed by the cited results sections by key question. This will be consolidated for the published article version of the report. |
| 7 | P. 28, Attention/Concentration paragraph, last line can read "....OR PTSD was not consistently associated with outcomes." | This change has been made. |
| 7 | P. 28, Key Question 1 paragraph, do not spell out neuropsychological test names. | This change has been made. |
| 7 | P. 28, last paragraph, "forensic" mentioned a couple of times – define what exactly this setting is. | This change has been made. |
| 7 | P. 29, first paragraph, indicate direction of associations; do not spell out LOC, PTA | This change has been made. |
| 7 | P. 29, Key Question 1 paragraph (here the 9 studies are cited, very helpful!); , do not spell out neuropsychological test names. | This change has been made. |

| Reviewer | Comment | Response |
|---|---|---|
| 7 | P. 29, 30 Key Question 2 paragraphs for each page, can say C&P instead of spelling it out; on p. 30, no need to define what a C&P evaluation is here, define it when first introduced | This change has been made. |
| 7 | P. 30 Effort/Motivation paragraph – regarding "with mTBI," see comment #41 | This change has been made. |
| 7 | P. 30, Key Question 2 paragraph, see comments #56, 58 | This change has been made. |
| 7 | P. 31, Key Question 1 paragraph, do not spell out neuropsychological test names. | This change has been made. |
| 7 | P. 31, Key Question 1 paragraph: There is discussion about "non-mTBI" participants – are these participants who never experienced a TBI (non-mTBI history) or who do not currently have mTBI (symptoms resolved?) | This has been clarified |
| 7 | P. 31, Key Question 2 paragraph: compensation and pension evaluation can be abbreviated | This change has been made. |
| 7 | P. 31, Self-reported Cognitive Problems paragraph. I'm wondering if "service connection" should be considered a "risk factor," as it's really a proxy for a disabling injury that was sustained or aggravated during military service. The point is taken that "service connection" is a short-hand for the latter, so this might be a matter of semantics. | Agreed, and this is how it is described in the primary study. |
| 7 | P. 31 – last word – instead of saying "control," say "control group." | This change has been made. |
| 7 | P. 32 – summary of Physical health results first paragraph – it would be helpful to cite the 16 studies here. | We are providing summary paragraphs without citations for each section, which are followed by the cited results sections by key question. This will be consolidated for the published article version of the report. |
| 7 | P. 32 – summary of Physical health results first paragraph – to be consistent, remove dashes from time-since-injury. | This change has been made. |
| 7 | P. 32 – second from last paragraph, no need to spell out NSI – already introduced. | This change has been made. |
| 7 | P. 33 – Table 3 – first row, similar to comment 63, "referral to neurology clinic for headaches" is listed as a risk factor, but is likely a proxy for headache severity/frequency. Again, this might just be a matter of semantics and readers will understand the implication. Without reviewing the article, not sure if any specifics were given for why a patient might be referred to a neurology clinic, so I understand that this might be the only unit of measurement. | Agreed—and this is how it was described in the primary study. |
| 7 | P.33 – Table 3 – some articles from JRRD 49(7) would be relevant here (if you increase the time frame of your search) | We have added these articles. |
| 7 | P. 34 – First paragraph – when describing the pain level scale, please provide anchors, 0 (no pain at all?) to 10 (very severe pain?) scale. | This change has been made. |

| Reviewer | Comment | Response |
|---|---|---|
| 7 | P. 34 – first paragraph for "Headaches," last line about referral to neurology clinic for headaches, see comment #68. | Noted. |
| 7 | P. 34 – Key Question 1 paragraph – here, the 9 studies being alluded to are actually cited (good!). Can also just say "NSI" here, no need to spell it out. | This change has been made. |
| 7 | P. 34 – Key Question 2 paragraph: Provide more detail in the first sentence – describe all groups being compared | This change has been made. |
| 7 | P. 34 – Key Question 2 paragraph, last sentence – see comment #68. | Noted. |
| 7 | P. 35 – "Vision" paragraph: cite the one study being discussed | We are providing summary paragraphs without citations for each section, which are followed by the cited results sections by key question. This will be consolidated for the published article version of the report. |
| 7 | P. 36 – "Nausea/Appetite" first paragraph - cite the specific studies you highlight, such as the study describing mild to moderate effects of mTBI population, PTSD studies, mixed results study | We are providing summary paragraphs without citations for each section, which are followed by the cited results sections by key question. This will be consolidated for the published article version of the report. |
| 7 | PP. 36-37 –Summary of Mental Health Results section – cite the studies where you describe 20 studies, two studies, PTSD, alcohol abuse, etc. | We are providing summary paragraphs without citations for each section, which are followed by the cited results sections by key question. This will be consolidated for the published article version of the report. |
| 7 | P. 38, Table 4, see comment #68 | Noted. |
| 7 | For the PTSD sections, 17 studies are alluded to in the first paragraph, and then alluded to again in the Key Question paragraph, and then cited. Just make sure there is consistency between the sections throughout the report in terms of when you cite. | Noted. |
| 7 | P. 39 - for Key Question 2, could you add specifics? For example, for study #27, what was the association between the PCL re-experiencing cluster and blast-exposure? | This change has been made. |
| 7 | P. 39 – For the anxiety paragraph, cite the studies that are being alluded to. | We are providing summary paragraphs without citations for each section, which are followed by the cited results sections by key question. This will be consolidated for the published article version of the report. |
| 7 | P. 39 – Key Question 1 – just say "NSI" | This change has been made. |
| 7 | P. 40 – Key Question 1 – abbreviations | This change has been made. |

148

| Reviewer | Comment | Response |
|---|---|---|
| 7 | P. 40 – Substance Use disorders first paragraph – cite studies alluded to | We are providing summary paragraphs without citations for each section, which are followed by the cited results sections by key question. This will be consolidated for the published article version of the report. |
| 7 | P. 40 –Suicide first paragraph - cite studies alluded to | We are providing summary paragraphs without citations for each section, which are followed by the cited results sections by key question. This will be consolidated for the published article version of the report. |
| 7 | P. 41 – Other Mental Health Outcomes first paragraph – cite studies alluded to | We are providing summary paragraphs without citations for each section, which are followed by the cited results sections by key question. This will be consolidated for the published article version of the report. |
| 7 | P. 41 – Other Mental Health Outcomes first paragraph – aren't "frustration" and "irritability" in the NSI affective cluster (e.g., Meterko et al., 2012, Journal of Head Trauma Rehabilitation, 27(1), 55-62 Psychometric assessment of the Neurobehavioral Symptom Inventory-22: the structure of persistent postconcussive symptoms following deployment-related mild traumatic brain injury among veterans.) | Yes, and we would consider these part of the mental health related outcomes section for this report. |
| 7 | P. 41 - Key Question 1 – abbreviations | This change has been made. |
| 7 | P. 41 - Key Question 1, second to last sentence – period before 12,20 citations. | This change has been made. |
| 7 | P. 41 – Summary of functional/social outcome results: cite studies alluded to | We are providing summary paragraphs without citations for each section, which are followed by the cited results sections by key question. This will be consolidated for the published article version of the report. |
| 7 | P. 41 – Summary of functional/social outcome results – make clear throughout the paragraph whether patients with mTBI, patients without mTBI, or results collapsed across both groups are being discussed. | This change has been made. |
| 7 | P. 43 – Sleep introduction paragraph – what are "positive neurological findings?" | This change has been made. |
| 7 | P. 43 – Sleep Key Question 1 – abbreviations | This change has been made. |
| 7 | P. 46 – In the "Results" paragraph: Throughout the paragraph, the word "obtaining" is used several times. I think a better word here would be "exhibiting." | This section has been removed and edited. |
| 7 | P. 46 –Key Question 1: Abbreviations | This section has been removed and edited. |
| 7 | P. 46 –Key Question 1: I found the first sentence difficult to follow – please add some additional punctuation and clarifying language. | This section has been removed and edited. |
| 7 | P. 46 – Key Question 2: the tense was different in this paragraph than in others. Use "exhibit" instead of "obtain." | This section has been removed and edited. |

| Reviewer | Comment | Response |
|---|---|---|
| 7 | P. 46 — Summary of service utilization/costs results: Please cite studies alluded to. | We are providing summary paragraphs without citations for each section, which are followed by the cited results sections by key question. This will be consolidated for the published article version of the report. |
| 7 | P. 48 – Key Question 1: Table X = Table 7? | This change has been made. |
| 7 | P. 50 – For mental health outcomes, it's acknowledged that PTSD is a focus for researchers, but I'm wondering if this section could be rounded out by also examining a few other mental health conditions that are typically of interest: depression, non-PTSD anxiety, and substance use disorders? As a starting point, Thomas W. McAllister has published on mild TBI in civilian populations and its after effects (e.g., cognitive, mental health conditions; Silver JM, McAllister TW, Arciniegas DB. Depression and cognitive complaints following mild traumatic brain injury. Am J Psychiatry. 2009; 166: 653-61.) | Agreed, and due to space limitations, we provided an expanded discussion of PTSD at the request of our stakeholders, but have not provided an expanded discussion of other outcomes, instead referring readers to other reviews and studies. |
| 7 | P. 50—3rd paragraph of the MH Outcomes section: instead of "causal factors," maybe use the term "event-related?" | This change has been made. |
| 7 | P. 50—in the "Not Surprisingly" paragraph, cite the "aforementioned" literature base. Also, in the last sentence of this paragraph, it might be more clear to say, "….related to mTBI versus other factors, such as those that are deployment-related, are not clear." | This change has been made. |
| 7 | P. 51—first partial paragraph at top, "When individuals experience the mTBI as traumatic," consider replacing "experience" with "perceive," since, by definition, the experience of mTBI is traumatic, at least physiologically/functionally. | This sentence has been clarified. |
| 7 | P. 51-first full paragraph, starting with "The results," I think more detail could be added here, such as citations, especially when you cite specific figures. Consider rewording the last sentence as: However, these high prevalence estimates may differ from results observed in civilian populations, as they may be related to unique deployment-related factors, such as combat, rather than, specifically, to the presence of mTBI. | This change has been made. |
| 7 | P. 51 – Imaging/biomarkers paragraph: cite the one study here. | We are providing summary paragraphs without citations for each section, which are followed by the cited results sections by key question. This will be consolidated for the published article version of the report. |
| 7 | P. 51 – "Although biomarkers" sentence: Do you mean "as prognostic tools among those with… "severe" TBI or with "moderate to severe" TBI? (not sure if severe was being used as a category, or if this was meant as "not mild." | This change has been made. |

| Reviewer | Comment | Response |
|---|---|---|
| 7 | P. 51 – "Although biomarkers" paragraph: after introducing chronic traumatic encephalopathy, put "(CTE)" | This change has been made. |
| 7 | P. 51 last paragraph, 2nd sentence, put "imaging" after "functional"; 5th sentence, use "DTI" instead of spelling it out; instead of "demonstrated" throughout this paragraph, use "observed;" Cite | This change has been made. |
| 7 | P. 52 – first paragraph, 2nd sentence; add "patients with" mTBI. | This change has been made. |
| 7 | P. 52 – first paragraph, 6th sentence, should be an "in" between "decreases memory" | This change has been made. |
| 7 | P. 52, first paragraph, 9th sentence, reword: differences between "individuals with mTBI" and "individuals without mTBI" or "individuals in the control group." | This change has been made. |
| 7 | P. 52, first paragraph, 9th sentence – reword, such as "fMRI studies found activation differences between individuals with mTBI and individuals in the control group during cognitive and behavioral tasks consistent with…." | This change has been made. |
| 7 | P. 52, first full paragraph, first sentence, reverse last two words so that it reads: mTBI neuroimaging; cite which studies found increased vs. decreased FA; instead of "controls," say "control participants." | This change has been made. |
| 7 | P. 54 – first paragraph, first sentence, say "universal" limitation (instead of across the board). | This has been re-worded. |
| 7 | P. 54 – first paragraph, what is the evidence that participants aren't blinded to study hypotheses? It's my sense that patients are told that the purpose of the study is to "examine differences," "observe," etc., and aren't informed about specific directional hypotheses until after study completion, if at all. | No studies reported that patients were blinded, and therefore we cannot assume that any were blinded. |
| 7 | P. 54 – second paragraph, 3rd-4th sentences; "wide variety of tools used to assess each outcome of interest." | This change has been made. |
| 7 | P. 54 –Conclusions, 2nd sentence, I would say, "The literature reviewed here," | This change has been made. |
| 7 | P. 54 – Conclusions, 4th sentence, instead of saying "negative outcomes," consider: "Though a significant portion of individuals who have experienced an mTBI report long-term mental and physical health symptoms" ….. "not significantly different from individuals who "did not experience mTBI" or "served as controls." | This section has been re-worded. |
| 7 | P. 54- Conclusions, 7th sentence, I would stay away from "outcomes," and say "self-reported symptoms," because we don't know whether symptoms/conditions are caused (i.e. an "outcome") by the mTBI. | This change has been made. |
| 7 | P. 54 –Conclusions, 8th sentence from last – instead of "do not have mTBI," I would say "who have not experienced mTBI" or "who do not have mTBI history" | This change has been made. |

| Reviewer | Comment | Response |
|---|---|---|
| 7 | P. 54 –Conclusions, 7th sentence from last, "instead of saying "is largely influenced by" I would say "can be accounted for" by other factors that are deployment-related, rather than…." | This change has been made. |
| 7 | P. 69 – Cameron et al., "five-difit", should be "five-digit" | This change has been made. |
| 7 | P. 72 – Hoge et al., "seeking starts" should be "seeing stars" | This change has been made. |
| 7 | P. 73- Luis et al., "loose" should be "lose" | This change has been made. |
| 7 | P. 87 & 96-Nelson et al. – why aren't the p-values listed? | We have listed results according to what was reported in the primary studies and have put labels used by study authors in quotes to indicate a direct quote in our tables. |
| 8 | Excellent that limitation of non-reporting of impaired subgroups is emphasized. | Noted. Thank you. |
| 8 | Text is somewhat repetitive and disorganized with regards to reporting of the conclusions reached. For example, conclusions are reported on p.13 within a paragraph on Literature Flow. | We have re-ordered the presentation of findings. |
| 8 | Presentation of results needs revision. Tables contain a great deal of text and no legends. Numbers are occasionally presented without units (e.g. p.18 Gordon et al; time since injury: 20.1 (weeks?)). Table 1 should include each study's outcome measures and preferably study hypothesis. It was good to see that effect sizes are reported in the tables in the appendices, but effect sizes are missing for most studies (if not reported, these can be calculated). Also, in cases where significance criteria have been corrected for multiple comparisons (e.g. Table 5), this should be indicated. | We have made these corrections to the table. For space reasons, we have presented some information in appendix tables rather than in text. We report the data as reported in the studies without calculating effect sizes when the authors did not provide this information; however, we are considering providing this calculated information in the article version of the report. |
| 8 | Discussion of imaging and biomarkers, p.51: it is mentioned twice that functional imaging studies have "failed" to show differences in performance along with differences in brain function, and this point would benefit from clarification. One explanation, supported by activation patterns, is that mTBI patients are able to accomplish similar test performance to uninjured controls through greater recruitment of neural resources. (e.g. McAllister, 2001, Neuroimage. 2001 Nov;14(5):1004-12.Differential working memory load effects after mild traumatic brain injury.) | We have moved all discussion of imaging results to the discussion due to searching limitations and refer readers to more comprehensive reviews of this literature. |
| 8 | p. 26 – Section title "Verbal and Old Learning" inappropriate as the tests described in this section measure vocabulary and knowledge, not learning (implies active learning and memory). | We have changed this title. |
| 8 | p. 26; paragraph 5: "…without mTBI on the RBANS Visuospatial/Constructional subscale." This sentence does not match information presented in table 1b for reference 33 | We have made sure these results are correct and consistent with the table. |

| Reviewer | Comment | Response |
|---|---|---|
| 8 | Within Appendix E, some information in the "comparison group description column" does not appear to describe a comparison group, but rather a covariate (e.g. PCL score). | Yes, this indicates continuous variables rather than comparison groups, and as such, correlation results are presented for these studies. |
| 8 | Readability comments: | Noted as below. |
| 8 | p.1 paragraph 1: "...and its associated post-concussion symptoms is..." should be "are" | Refers to mTBI, not the symptoms, therefore left as "is." |
| 8 | p. 1 paragraph 1: "...a TBI while deployed)." The parenthesis does not have a partner. | This change has been made. |
| 8 | p.1 paragraph 2 and p.8 paragraph 2: "...balance problems) beyond this time fame;" should be "frame" | This change has been made. |
| 8 | p. 1 paragraph 2: "...often require the attention from a range of health care professionals..." should remove "the" | This change has been made. |
| 8 | p.3 paragraph 4: "lengthly" should be "lengthy" | This change has been made. |
| 8 | p. 3 paragraph 5: "...Veteran/military participants without mTBI)." The parenthesis does not have a partner. | This change has been made. |
| 8 | p. 9 paragraph 6: "disruption of brain function (e.g. altered of consciousness...)" should be "alteration" | This change has been made. |
| 8 | p. 28 paragraph 4: "six studies reporting..." Should be "reported" | This change has been made. |
| 8 | p. 41 paragraph 3: "Axis 1" should be "Axis I" | This change has been made. |
| 8 | p. 54 paragraph 3: "...we excluded many studies which proported to study mTBI" should be "purported" | This change has been made. |
| 9 | The work of Drs Cockerham and Goodrich might be beneficial in the section on Vision as it addresses occult visual deficits in this patient population. This can often be conflated with self-reported complaints, as previously established mechanisms of assessment were deemed not sensitive in detecting these abnormalities. Additionally, as this data is prospectively collected at all Polytrauma sites, could this data be incorporated in the analyses. | We have reviewed this literature and though it provides important information related to vision outcomes, we did not find studies meeting our inclusion criteria for this report due to the populations examined. |
| 9 | Would also recommend additional references regarding TBI incidence—pg #8 Introduction. The point could be substantiated by and WHO data or CDC Data. | We have re-worked the introduction for the report. |

| Reviewer | Comment | Response |
|---|---|---|
| 10 | In a significant number of veterans and service members who have incurred a blast or non-blast related mTBI have lead to persistent or chronic post-concussion syndrome (PCS). Multiple studies have reported PCS-like symptoms among Veterans many years after mTBI. Agree that published studies to date has been unable to identify all the potential risk factors and a major causative role other than mTBI. ICD-10 and DSM-4 criteria have been established for diagnosing PCS and differ somewhat. There continues to be a lack of consensus regarding PCS, ICD-10 guidelines limit the symptoms to within 4 weeks of injury, while DSM-4 criteria requires symptom onset shortly after injury, but persistence at least 3 months. Despite these diagnostic guidelines, evidence suggests that symptoms can appear immediately, or weeks to months after the initial injury (Ryan et al.2006) and recent studies have reported PCS-like symptoms among Veterans many years after mTBI. (Scholten et al.2012). While these persistent symptoms are known to complicate return to work/duty and negatively affect quality of life, their trajectories and time courses are not understood and diagnosis remains challenging and relies mostly on self-report of complex symptomatology rather than objective, quantitative or biological measures. The reasons why people recover slowly or fail to recover fully from mTBIs is not known and there are no current methodologies for diagnosis or prognosis of PCS. Identifying the cognitive, clinical, and serum biomarkers that accurately diagnose veterans or service members with persistent symptoms is critical to our understanding of long-term outcomes in this patient population and needs to explored further. | We have expanded the discussion section to include some of these ideas. |
| 11 | This was a challenging area with limited available published studies. I would suggest plainly stating in the early overview section that there are no prospective randomized RCTs. | We have stated this in the executive summary and the body of the report. |
| 11 | The overview also seems somewhat contradictory when you report that imaging findings are of low strength of evidence yet your recommendations indicate that prospective studies should be designed to report imaging findings. | We have rearranged and clarified the imaging findings and recommendations. |

*Optional Dissemination and Implementation Questions*

**5. Are there any VA clinical performance measures, programs, quality improvement measures, patient care services, or conferences that will be directly affected by this report? If so, please provide detail.**

| 5 | There really is no new information here. Conclusions are consistent with other reviews. However, making this available to national Polytrauma calls or conferences, and Mental Health/PTSD calls and conferences would help reinforce these findings. | Noted. We plan to make the report findings available in a variety of formats, including VA intranet, a published article, presentation at a national neuropsychology conference, and through a VA cyber-seminar. We will consider how to expand the audience as you recommend. |

| Reviewer | Comment | Response |
|---|---|---|
| 6 | Yes. The results raise the question of the context in which mTBI may be best treated within VA. The results also have implications for compensation and pension decisions regarding mTBI. | Noted, though we caution our readers not to make strong inferences based on the low quality literature available for synthesis in this report. Relying on these report findings in conjunction with related research on civilian populations with mTBI will provide the strongest available foundation for such weighty decisions. |
| 7 | Because "time since injury" was cited throughout the document as being related to impairment, but also noted to be missing in many studies, I think it would be very important to capture this variable in national VA databases, such as the Comprehensive TBI Evaluation database. If this information is available in any DoD databases, like Defense Manpower Data Center (DMDC), then a data exchange between DoD and VA would benefit studies by having these data located in one central source, thus reducing the risk of error through patient self-report. | We have added this to the discussion. |
| 8 | Given the limited nature and low quality of literature, it is not possible to reach firm conclusions. There is nothing to be implemented at this time. | Noted, and we encourage readers of this report to consider the results in conjunction with findings from civilian literature in order to make conclusions based on the best available evidence. |
| 9 | Vision Screening in the Inpatient/Polytrauma Units might be affected. | Noted. |
| 10 | Yes. Polytrauma/ TBI System of Care. | Noted. |
| 11 | Polytrauma System of Care, can be disseminated on one of the national calls and emailing providers with link to report. | Noted. |
| **6. Please provide any recommendations on how this report can be revised to more directly address or assist implementation needs.** | | |
| 1 | You might consider adding review of any studies that looked at multiple mTBI's. It is a common "complication" Also, on page 1, I'd suggest clearly delineating the difference between cognitive performance and symptom complaints. While it's true that the literature suggests complete cognitive performance recovery by 3 months (or even 7 days in sports literature), there is a difference between performance and symptoms. Furthermore, the civilian literature suggests that PCS symptoms in fact do not *persist* (See Meares et al) and such the use of the term 'persist' may be incorrect. "Presence" may be more accurate. | We have made these changes throughout the report. |
| 5 | There is no "So What" section. However, one could potentially make the suggestion that since outcomes do not differ following mTBI, that all the DoD/VHA time, energy, and attention devoted to this matter may be a less than ideal use of resources. For example: Do we really need to continue to screen for mTBI? Are the required Comprehensive TBI Evaluations following a positive TBI screen, really needed and a good use of resources? | Noted, and we have expanded our discussion of these points in the report. |

| Reviewer | Comment | Response |
|---|---|---|
| 5 | Are there better ways to meet the needs of those symptomatic returning service members and veterans than focusing on mTBI, when mTBI does not appear to be the factor explaining the symptoms and problems? | Noted, and we have expanded our discussion of this point in the report. |
| 6 | No recommendations. This is a thorough report with well-reasoned conclusions. | Noted. Thank you. |
| 7 | This report indicates that many of the mTBI studies performed with service members and Veterans are methodologically limited and provide low strength evidence. Because implementation should be based on strong evidence, it doesn't appear that this report should make any health services related recommendations on implementation, but should recommend that VA leaders prioritize research funding to ensure high quality research, and develop mechanisms (e.g., databases, standard communications between DoD and VA) that assist researchers in obtaining reliable data. | We agree that ideally, recommendations should be made based on strong evidence. However, in the absence of strong evidence, then the best available evidence should be the basis on which treatment and policy decisions are made. We have made cautious recommendations consistent with the best available evidence for treatment and policy as well as making strong recommendations for further high quality research as you suggest. |
| 8 | Readability and typographical errors should be addressed. Presentation of results should be revised. Consider other data presentation modes in addition to tables. Imaging and biomarkers could possibly be removed and examined in a separate report with selection criteria that are more appropriate for these kinds of studies. | Noted, and we have incorporated your suggested edits. |
| 10 | The current focus in the TBI clinics is the CHRONIC effects of mTBI 3-10 years post injury with retained sequelae of the initial injury which does not completely follow the recovery pattern of the civilian mTBI population. In the civilian population the symptoms are transient and self-limiting, with apparent full recovery occurring from minutes to several weeks following injury (Levin et al., 1997) which is distinct from our veteran/service member population who have persistent symptoms and/or functional limitations (Iverson et al., 2006; Ruff et al., 1996). There needs to be further investigation into the etiology and treatment of these chronic/persistent PCS symptoms. | We agree and have expanded our discussion of treatment implications. |
| | **7. Please provide us with contact details of any additional individuals/stakeholders who should be made aware of this report.** | |
| 5 | DCoE, DVBIC, VBA? | Noted. |
| 6 | No specific recommendations other than VA polytrauma staff. | Noted. |
| 7 | HSR&D/QUERI/RR&D leaders responsible for prioritizing funding, inclusive of and addition to:<br>David X. Cifu, MD<br>Nina A. Sayer, PhD<br>Joel Scholten, MD<br>Doug Bidelspach, MPT<br>VA TBI/Polytrauma Clinic Directors | Noted. |

| Reviewer | Comment | Response |
|---|---|---|
| 8 | Katherine Helmick, Deputy Director, Defense and Veterans Brain Injury Center katherine.helmick@tma.osd.mil | Noted. |
| 10 | The following stakeholders should made aware of this report: VHA Polytrauma System of Care which include Polytrauma Rehabilitation Centers (PRC),Polytrauma Transitional Rehabilitation Programs (PTRP), Polytrauma Network Site (PNS), Polytrauma Support Clinic Team (PSCT), and Polytrauma Point of Contact (PPOC). In addition the Military Heath System's TBI clinics, Defense and Veterans Brain Injury Center (DVBIC) and National Intrepid Center of Excellence (NICoE) satellite TBI clinics. | Noted. |